Intradiscal Therapy
Chymopapain or Collagenase

INTRADISCAL THERAPY
Chymopapain or Collagenase

MARK D. BROWN, M.D., Ph.D.

Professor of Orthopaedics and Rehabilitation and Neurological Surgery
University of Miami School of Medicine
Miami, Florida

Illustrated by
Leona M. Allison

YEAR BOOK MEDICAL PUBLISHERS, INC.
CHICAGO • LONDON

Library of Congress Cataloging in Publication Data

Brown, Mark D.
   "Intradiscal therapy chymopapain or collagenase."

   Bibliography: p.
   1. Intervertebral disk—Hernia—Chemotherapy.
2. Chymopapain—Therapeutic use.   3. Collagenases—
Therapeutic use.   4. Injections, Intradiscal.
I. Title.   [DNLM: 1. Peptide peptidohydrolases—
Therapeutic use.   2. Clostridiopeptidase A—
Therapeutic use.   3. Intervertebral disk
displacement—Drug therapy.   WE 740 B879i]
RD771.I6B76   1983   617'.56061   83-1188
ISBN 0-8151-1282-3

*This book is dedicated to the patients with disc herniation
who participated in the early investigations
of intradiscal therapy. They risked placebo injections
and prolonged suffering so that others might benefit
from what was learned.*

Table of Contents

Foreword

INTRADISCAL THERAPY for the treatment of herniation of the nucleus pulposis represents a major breakthrough in the treatment of this common affliction. The release of chymopapain for general use makes this book most timely. Dr. Brown has summarized the total experience with the enzyme thus far. This work should be read by every surgeon who contemplates performing chemonucleolysis.

The history of chymopapain given in the first chapter is interesting reading and should be part of the disc surgeon's fund of knowledge. Perhaps the most important is the chapter dealing with the prevention of anaphylaxis. This is the complication most feared. It can, however, be controlled if proper precautions are used.

The technique of injection will differ somewhat between hospitals, depending on the particular radiographic machinery available. The surgeon is admonished to insist on good fluoroscopic equipment right from the start. Placing the needle into the proper area of the disc is often difficult, especially at L-5. Poor needle placement is a common reason for failure to obtain a satisfactory clinical result.

The report on the present status of collagenase will be of great interest to all who are planning to use intradiscal therapy. Experience with collagenase is far less than with chymopapain, but collagenase is a very promising drug. I am aware of no one other than Dr. Brown who has had personal experience in the clinical use of both chymopapain and collagenase, so he is eminently qualified to write on the subject.

I believe we are at the dawn of a new era in disc surgery. In the coming years, chemical discolysis will far exceed surgical removal in number of cases of classical disc herniation treated. Other as yet unexplored conditions such as painful disc degeneration without sciatica may be found to respond to intradiscal therapy. Suffice it to say, those of us involved in the treatment of disc disease can look forward to a fascinating decade.

L. L. WILTSE, M. D.

Preface

DESCRIBING THE FIRST TEN PATIENTS treated in 1963 by intradiscal injection of chymopapain, Lyman Smith wrote, "A new method of treatment for the chronic, recurring, and puzzling condition of herniation of the nucleus pulposus needs time and large numbers of patients before an adequate evaluation can be made." Twenty years later, 40,000 patients have been treated by chemonucleolysis with chymopapain, and vast amounts of data and controversy concerning both the procedure and the drug have been generated.

An alternative enzyme, collagenase, has also been tested and is in the third phase of clinical trials. A comparison of the pharmacology and clinical action of these two agents is now available.

The purpose of this book is to summarize and correlate information on these two enzymes in the treatment of herniated discs so that orthopedists, neurosurgeons, neurologists, radiologists, anesthesiologists, auxiliary health personnel, and health care planners can make rational decisions as to their use.

After reviewing the literature on chemonucleolysis, conducting clinical trials with both chymopapain and collagenase, and observing the action of both enzymes in the laboratory, I began this book by asking myself: If I personally had a disabling disc displacement of the lumbar spine that had not improved with time and/or conservative care, would I undergo chemonucleolysis instead of laminectomy? If so, which enzyme would I choose? My answer to the first question—based on the extensive data on chymopapain's nature, benefits, and risks—is an unqualified yes! I cannot answer the second question because all the data on collagenase are not yet available. However, it is beneficial for the patient to have available two distinctly different enzymes, should a second injection be necessary. Reinjection with chymopapain is currently not advocated because of potential allergenicity.

Ultimately, a better enzyme than either chymopapain or collagenase will be discovered. The qualities that this new drug should have and its potential effects on patient care are discussed in the final chapter of this book.

MARK D. BROWN

Acknowledgments

WITHOUT THE DEDICATION and sincerity of the following people, this book would not have been completed: M. Patricia Brown, R.N. (moral support, typing), Gloria Coutts (typing and other secretarial work), Leona Allison (medical illustration), Janet Tompkins, R.N. (bibliography and proofreading), Hilda Lo, Ph.D. (electron microscopy), Octavio Martinez, Ph.D. and Maria Ramos (biochemistry), Björn Rydevik, M.D. (effects of chymopapain and collagenase on nerve tissue), John Bromley, M.D. (Nucleolysin double-blind study), LeWayne Stromberg, M.D. (Discase triple-blind study), Rob Fraser, M.D. (Discase Australian double-blind study), Eugene Nordby, M.D. (Chymodiactin double-blind study), John McCulloch, M.D. (anaphylaxis experience), Leon Wiltse, M.D. (clinical experience and disc height restoration), Eugene Coin, M.D. (CAT scans before and after collagenase), Arthur Naylor, M.D. (unpublished biochemistry data, chymopapain), Alf Nachemson, M.D. (unpublished data, prospective clinical study), Edwin Wegman, Harold Stern, Ph.D., and Judy Hirst, Ph.D. (Advance Biofactures Corporation, manufacturers of Nucleolysin), James Simmons, M.D. (information on Chemolase, chymopapain manufactured by OrthoTex Labs), and, most important—Anthony F. DePalma, M.D., for his vision and inspiration to continue a lifetime of clinically applied research. Finally, I would like to acknowledge Ed Wickland, Editorial Director of Year Book Medical Publishers, for his perception of the importance and timeliness of this information, and the staff at Year Book, Fran Perveiler, Editing Supervisor, Sharon Pepping, Project Manager, Lois Smit, Senior Copy Editor, and Shirley Taylor, Proofroom Supervisor, for their hard work. Because of the efforts of this team, accurate and very current information, which will be of help to so many patients, has been published with a speed almost unparalleled in medical book publishing.

1 / History of Chemonucleolysis

In 1959, Carl Hirsch[1] ended a paper on the pathology of low back pain with the suggestion that "either we will have to find methods by which discs can recover biologically and we will have to improve the nutritional mechanism, which does not seem to lie within our reach, or we will have to find methods by which the deterioration can rapidly pass the stage at which a mechanical disorder causes pain. Sooner or later a substance may be found by which a degenerated disc could be transformed to dense connective tissue. It might be possible to create a chondrolytic enzyme that, injected into a disc, would cause a connective tissue reaction."

Whereas Hirsch envisioned an enzyme that would induce a fibrotic reaction and thus heal and stabilize the degenerated intervertebral disc, Lyman Smith wanted to develop a chemical that would dissolve the herniated disc that causes leg pain by compressing spinal nerves. In 1963, he described the pharmacology of such a chondrolytic enzyme.[2] The enzyme was chymopapain, a crystalline fraction of papaya latex from the fruit of the papaya plant; and it was found to be effective in dissolving the nucleus pulposus of the intervertebral disc in normal rabbits.

EARLY HISTORY

The early history of chemical dissolution of the nucleus pulposus parallels the discovery and development of the enzyme chymopapain. However, before tracing the development of chymopapain, it is worthwhile to review the pathophysiology of disc degeneration and disc herniation. Keep in mind that 20 years of experience with chymopapain has helped us to understand both the pathophysiology of disc displacement and the natural history of this common disorder.

PATHOPHYSIOLOGY OF THE INTERVERTEBRAL DISC

The pathophysiology of disc degeneration was documented in the medical literature around the time that chymopapain was being developed. However, the natural history of symptoms related to this disorder became more apparent in the ensuing 20 years, when controlled trials for treatment were performed.

It was known that the intervertebral disc was devoid of blood and depended upon passive diffusion for nutrition.[3] There was some speculation that the cells responsible for maintaining the matrix of the disc were in a precarious position due to the highly avascular nature of the structure, and that faulty nutrition of these cells was somehow related to their demise and the subsequent degeneration of the disc matrix.[4]

It was also known that there were no sensory nerve endings in the disc itself.[5] Free and complex nerve endings had been discovered in the longitudinal ligaments and extreme peripheral layers of the annulus fibrosus; nerve endings were also associated with the vascular loops in the subchondral bony end plate of the intervertebral disc.

The existing theory concerning the normal function of the intervertebral disc was that forces applied to the spine were distributed by the nucleus pulposus to place tension on the surrounding annulus fibrosus.[6] It was theorized that the nucleus pulposus functioned as a hydrostatic ball bearing and that its matrix was composed of water-binding protein polysaccharide molecules with randomly dispersed and intimately associated collagen fibers.[7]

Disc degeneration was known to be an ubiquitous phenomenon, the incidence of which increased with aging. Disc disease is defined as a painful and/or disabling result of such degeneration, which begins with loss of the gel-like structure of the nucleus pulposus, which results in compression of the annulus fibrosus. The fibroblasts in the annulus fibrosus, exposed to compression rather than tension, produce cartilage between the lamellar fibers. Concentric fissures result, followed by radial tears through the annulus fibrosus.[8]

Electron microscopic examination of discs[9] at various ages shows that young nucleus pulposus contains randomly dispersed collagen fibers bound to protein polysaccharides. With aging, the protein polysaccharide in the nucleus pulposus matrix decreases, and the collagen appears more prominent in electron microscopic studies because the periodic bands of collagen fibers are not obscured by the protein polysaccharides.

Biochemical data[10] show that, with aging, there is a decrease in the total water content of the nucleus pulposus, associated with a decrease in the total amount and type of protein polysaccharides, and a relative increase in the collagen content of the disc. Physiologically, there is a decrease in the permeability of the tissue matrix and in the ability of the disc to withstand load, related to the decrease in protein polysaccharide of the nucleus pulposus.

The theoretical mechanism of how disc degeneration results in symptomatic disc disease is that genetically modulated biochemical events cause the disc matrix proteoglycans to lose their water-binding capacity. Since the proteoglycans are responsible for the normal weight-bearing characteristics of the disc, loss of function in these macromolecules renders the nucleus pulposus less capable of withstanding loads. The annulus not only is subjected to abnormal compressive loads (normally it functions under tension) but also becomes susceptible to radial tears within the range of physiologic torsion strains. When radial tears occur in the annulus fibrosus, the nucleus pulposus may herniate through these tears. When the herniated nucleus pulposus presses on the peripheral layers of the annulus fibrosus and longitudinal ligaments containing the nerve endings, back pain may result. Further prolapse or extrusion of nuclear material may compress and irritate the spinal nerve roots and cause leg pain. John Charnley[11] demonstrated that pressures of a swelling nucleus pulposus could reach 300 mm Hg, well above the systemic arterial pressure, which could account for the marked tension noted on the nerve root at laminectomy for removal of a pain-producing herniated disc.

Chronic low back pain was theorized to be secondary to mechanical instability of the motion segment unit, resulting from the poor weight-bearing ability of the degenerated intervertebral disc.[12]

It was also theorized that the byproducts of tissue breakdown in the nucleus pulposus, leaking through cracks in the vertebral body end plates or tears in the annulus fibrosus, produced a direct inflammation of the nerves or an indirect inflammation through a local autoimmune reaction.[13]

CHYMOPAPAIN, THE IDEAL ENZYME

Using the theories of disc degeneration and disc displacement at the end of the 1950s, Lyman Smith conceptualized that it would be possible to chemically dissolve herniated discs.

In 1956, Lewis Thomas[14] showed that, if rabbits were injected intravenously with crude papain, their ears would collapse within 4 hours, due to a depletion of the mucoid portion of the ear cartilage matrix. If a large amount of papain was injected, the matrix of other cartilaginous tissues, including joint cartilage, the epiphyseal growth plate, and tracheal and bronchial cartilage, was also affected. The ears resumed their normal shape with time, and there was a coincidental restoration of the basophilic chondroid matrix. Thomas could not reproduce these results with activated crystalline papain, but it was later determined that *in*activated crystalline papain would produce the same results.[15] It seemed that activated enzyme reacted with the plasma proteins before arriving at the ear cartilage matrix, whereas the inactivated enzyme would bypass the serum proteins and selectively bind to cartilage matrix, thereby becoming activated and able to lyse the proteoglycans of the cartilage. Several other investigators have shown that the papain selectively hydrolyzes the protein core of the acid mucopolysaccharide molecule, depletes the cartilage matrix of its basophilic staining character, releases chondroitin sulfate into the circulation, and causes structural changes in the ear cartilage.[16]

In his quest for a chemical that could remove herniated discs rich in protein polysaccharides, Smith settled on a twice-crystallized fraction of papaya latex called chymopapain, whose activity was based on the amounts of protein released from cartilage powder. He tested the dose in rabbit lumbar intervertebral discs and found that the nucleus pulposus was dissolved according to the amount of chymopapain injected. The action of the enzyme was selective for the nucleus pulposus, and only large doses caused some change in the annulus fibrosus. As little as .05 mg per disc caused disc narrowing visible on x-ray, whereas 10 mg per disc—when injected into three or four discs—could produce lethal hemorrhage in the gastrointestinal tract, abdominal cavity, and lungs.

Smith noted that chymopapain was highly toxic when injected intrathecally in rabbits. Doses as small as 0.0625 mg per kilogram in a volume as small as 1 ml produced paralysis and death. These changes occurred from disruption of the bonds between the endothelial cells in the capillaries of the pia-arachnoid membranes, which resulted in intrathecal hemorrhage. However, chymopapain did not have any immediate effect on the functional conduction of electrical impulses when it was placed on frog and rabbit sciatic nerves. Although Smith tested other enzymes, chymopapain turned out to be the most selective for chemically removing nucleus pulposus.

Nothing is new under the sun, and it is interesting that Ball[17] reported on a new treatment of ganglion in 1940 by the injection of a proteolytic enzyme called caroid, a crude papaya extract. Ball discovered that the enzyme would liquefy the gelatinous (protein-polysaccharide-rich) contents of the ganglion within 30 minutes after injection and make it easy to aspirate the contents of the ganglion with a needle and syringe. The use of the papaya enzyme in humans for dissolving proteoglycans had already been tried.

Incidentally, not only had papaya enzyme been used in humans to dissolve proteoglycans, but also Henry Feffer had had extensive experience in the treatment of low back and sciatic pain by injectioning hydrocortisone into degenerated intervertebral discs.[18] Feffer performed "nucleograms," later to be called discograms, before the intradiscal injection of hydrocortisone. Sixty-seven percent of the patients that he treated had rapid remission of symptoms; 33% failed to respond. His rationale was based on the supposition that there was an inflammatory process that resulted from the degenerated disc.

CLINICAL TRIALS OF CHYMOPAPAIN

Having established the fact that chymopapain could dissolve the nucleus pulposus in rabbits without injuring surrounding epidural tissues, Smith treated 22 dogs with hindquarters paralyzed from herniated intervertebral discs. Fourteen had reversal of their hind-limb paralysis and were able to stand or walk. Six failed to improve, and postmortem examination showed herniation of discs at levels that were not injected. More important, at autopsy there were no adverse effects that could be attributed to intradiscal injection of the enzyme. One dog had degeneration of the spinal cord below the lesion, and one dog was not accounted for.

Between July 11 and August 19, 1963, Smith[19] treated his first 10 patients with "incapacitating sciatica" by intradiscal injection of chymopapain. His original patient selection was confused by the fact that six of the 10 patients had previously undergone laminectomy without relief of symptoms. He utilized a posterior lateral approach to the disc as described by Erlacher,[20] where the needle is passed just lateral to the dura, but within the bony spinal canal, and into the center of the disc (Plate 1). A discogram was performed with sodium diatrizoate (Hypaque) prior to the chymopapain injection. There was a fascinating observation that seven of the 10 patients had relief of leg and back pain within 6 to 18 hours after injection. Within 4 to 8 days following injection, all 10 patients showed narrowing of the disc space on x-rays—objective evidence that chymopapain was acting on the disc.

After injection, patients complained of increased back pain, lasting for a week to 10 days, which Smith attributed to settling of the disc space and resultant stress on the articular facets. Of the 3 patients who failed to respond to treatment, one was found to have an extruded fragment of disc when operated on within 3 weeks of injection.

Encouraged by his early results between September 1963 and January 1964, Smith injected 30 more patients with chymopapain in collaboration with Joseph E. Brown of St. Luke's Hospital in Cleveland. Thus began Phase I in the clinical testing of chymopapain to determine the appropriate dosage, response, and risks in treating patients with herniated discs.

Results in Dogs With Disc Disease

Later in 1964, Saunders[21] reported the results of chymopapain in the treatment of canine intervertebral disc syndrome. Seventy-five dogs with paralyzed hindquarters were injected; within 8 to 12 days after injection, 39 were walking, 14 had improved, 16 showed no improvement, and 6 had died. Autopsy showed various forms of advanced pathologic conditions, but no deleterious effects from the enzyme. Saunders pointed out in this study that chymopapain should *not* be reconstituted with water containing preservatives because they inactivated the enzymes. He also cautioned against the use of x-ray contrast media as a diluent for fear of inactivating the enzyme. The latter fear was later found to be unwarranted; actually, the action of the enzyme may be enhanced by contrast dye.

Initial Clinical Trial in Humans

In October 1965, Smith and Brown presented the results of their initial clinical trials to the British Orthopaedic Association in London. The paper documenting these results appeared in the *Journal of Bone and Joint Surgery* in 1967.[22] They treated 75 patients, 22 of whom had undergone previous laminectomy. The last 32 patients in this series were injected via a lateral approach to the disc developed by Edholm et al.[23] (see Plate 1). Because this approach avoids penetration of the dura altogether (and therefore the inadvertent injection of chymopapain into the subarachnoid space) the complication of headaches is minimized.

Clinical Course

Following injection of chymopapain, patients experienced dramatic relief of leg pain within 24 hours. The decrease in leg pain was incomplete and usually improved over the next 4 to 6 weeks to complete recovery.

Thirty-nine percent of the 75 patients had severe muscle spasms and increased back pain, usually within 6 to 8 hours after injection and lasting from 12 to 24 hours. However, 12 out of the 75 patients had no appreciable back pain after injection. Most had excellent relief of symptoms within 4 weeks.

Smith and Brown's original compilation of results showed that 86% of 53 patients *without* previous spinal surgery had a good result, with no back or leg pain, and were able to participate in their usual occupational and recreational activities. Six of the 75 patients had poor results, and only one was made worse by the treatment.

Problems Encountered

Neural toxicity.—In case 37 of Smith and Brown's series, 5 days after a myelogram in which 5 ml of Pantopaque was left in the subarachnoid space, the patient underwent discography by the posterolateral approach at three levels in the lumbar spine. There was difficulty penetrating the fifth lumbar space, and multiple dural punctures were made. A total of 30 mg of chymopapain, 10 mg per disc, was injected. Although the patient's leg pain disappeared within 6 hours, he experienced severe back and abdominal pain. Over the next 5 days he had an acute abdominal crisis, and on the tenth day he was paraplegic. At laminectomy (from the fourth thoracic to the fifth lumbar vertebra), severe hemorrhagic arachnoiditis was noted at the tenth thoracic level, although the third, fourth, and fifth lumbar intervertebral discs had been injected.

Repeated studies on the toxicity of chymopapain were performed by intrathecal and epidural injections in rabbits, cats, and dogs. From these studies, Garvin and his colleagues[24] concluded that the paraplegia in Smith and Brown's Case 37 was secondary to a subarachnoid mixture of Pantopaque and blood from the myelogram. Garvin stated that, if the subarachnoid hemorrhage had been caused by chymopapain, the patient would have immediately exhibited symptoms of increased intracranial pressure, a phenomenon noted in animals following intrathecal injection of chymopapain. Since previous animal studies with Pantopaque and blood mixed in the subarachnoid space had resulted in arachnoiditis,[25] it was concluded that the large amount of retained Pantopaque and subsequently induced hemorrhage from difficult transdural needle placement caused the arachnoiditis leading to paraplegia. Regardless of what occurred in this case, the animal studies did show that the intrathecal injection of chymopapain should be avoided.

MISDIAGNOSIS.—Another complication was due primarily to failure of diagnosis. A patient was injected with 10 mg of chymopapain into the sixth cervical disc following discography, but without prior myelography or spinal fluid analysis. Pain was relieved for 2 weeks but subsequently recurred. Six weeks after injection, the patient developed a Brown-Séquard syndrome. Three subsequent laminectomies were required before an adequate biopsy specimen could be obtained and malignant hemangioendothelioma diagnosed.

Subsequent thorough scrutiny of this case has led to the conclusion that the patient suffered from a rare malignant tumor in the cervical spinal cord meninges and coincidental cervical disc disease. However, on the basis of this case, it was deemed appropriate to limit the use of chymopapain to lumbar disc disease in all subsequent trials, and to confirm the diagnosis by myelogram.

SENSITIVITY REACTIONS.—The third complication encountered in Smith and Brown's original series occurred in Case 27 following discography. Chymopapain (10 mg) was injected into the fourth lumbar level and 7 mg into the fifth lumbar level. Three weeks later, a second dose of 9 mg was injected into the fourth and fifth lumbar discs. The patient had a generalized systemic reaction with a dramatic fall in blood pressure and a cutaneous reaction. Treatment with steroids and epinephrine resulted in recovery within the hour. No antibodies against chymopapain were detected in this patient's sera 3 weeks after injection.

From previous guinea pig studies, it was concluded that chymopapain was a relatively poor antigen. Anaphylaxis was thought to have resulted from the Hypaque (a substance known to be potentially allergenic) used during discography.

Another patient developed giant urticaria 10 days after injection. Although this particular complication was not attributed to chymopapain, it subsequently became evident that a number of patients had been previously sensitized to papaya enzyme.

Other "problems."—Another patient had symptoms of a low-grade disc space infection after injection, but this was never really proved. In yet another patient, 7 months after injection of 8 mg of chymopapain into the L-4 disc, a myelogram showed a blockage at the L4-5 level. A laminectomy revealed a small area of "filmy arachnoiditis" at the fifth lumbar level. The patient had some relief of back pain, but the evidence that chymopapain had caused the arachnoiditis was not convincing. This was probably a case of central disc displacement and/or spinal stenosis. A preinjection myelogram might have eliminated this patient as a candidate for injection.

Conclusions

The lesson learned from Smith's original clinical trials was that patients with no previous surgery who had a primary complaint of leg pain were excellent candidates for the procedure (Table 1–1). The injection should be performed via the lateral route proposed by Edholm,[23] thus avoiding dural penetration. Although chymopapain did not seem to have a deleterious effect on surrounding tissue, it was potentially dangerous to inject it intrathecally; it seemed to be allergenic; and it was deemed appropriate to limit its use to the lumbar spine following thorough diagnosis, including a myelogram and cerebral spinal fluid analysis.

EARLY CRITICISM AND CONTROVERSY REGARDING CHYMOPAPAIN AND CHEMONUCLEOLYSIS

Prior to the publication of Smith and Brown's article, Normal Shealy, a neurosurgeon involved in the care of one of Smith and Brown's patients, reported on the case.[26]

A 50-year-old man had pain relief for several weeks after a 10-mg injection of chymopapain into the sixth cervical disc. Two months later, he developed intermittent weakness in his right hand. A cervical myelogram showed a large extramedullary mass at C6-7. The cerebral spinal fluid protein level was 400 mg%. A laminectomy was performed between C-6 and T-1 and the dura was opened; a large reddish mass,

TABLE 1–1.—Results of Clinical Trial of Chymopapain in Patients With No Previous Surgery, 1963–1969

INVESTIGATOR	NO. OF PATIENTS	Good	RESULTS Fair	Poor
L. Smith	112	99	4	9
P. Day	86	77	8	1
Total	198	176 (88%)	12 (7%)	10 (5%)

presumed to be a pseudoaneurysm, was noted over the C6-7 interspace. Postoperatively, the patient had a wound infection, which healed by open treatment and secondary granulation. Three months following the chymopapain injection, the patient was taken back to the operating room, and a second biopsy revealed vascularized granulation tissue. The patient's condition gradually worsened, and 5 months after injection the wound was explored for the third time and diagnosis of invasive hemangioendothelioma was made by biopsy.

Shealy points out that, had a myelogram been performed on this patient, the disc would not have been injected unnecessarily. He stated that it was a fallacy to treat patients on the basis of discography alone and quoted the work of Holt, who showed that 138 out of 148 cervical discograms in asymptomatic subjects were abnormal.[27] Shealy also points out the dangers of epidural steroid injections for back and leg pain before ruling out such conditions as disc space infection.

CONFUSING DATA REGARDING TOXICITY

Shealy also addressed the problem of neural toxicity specific to chymopapain.[28] Forty-two adult cats had therapeutic concentrations of chymopapain injected into the dura, the brain, the adventitia of the carotid artery, the subarachnoid space, and the liver and/or spleen. One laminectomy was performed and the enzyme dripped onto the dura. After two months, two animals showed chronic inflammation and necrosis of nerve and muscle in the thoracic epidural space. One had a thickened arachnoid and another, a tremendous epidural foreign body granulomatous reaction. Wherever chymopapain was injected, there was tissue necrosis and destruction of the walls of small blood vessels. Arachnoidal thickening was observed in four of eight animals who survived epidural injection from 1 to 4 months. Shealy concluded that chymopapain produced a chronic foreign-body granulomatous inflammation or necrosis when injected into the epidural space.

Subsequent review of Shealy's slides by Ian MacNab[29] allegedly showed foreign-body granulation secondary to birefringent crystals, consistent with talc granulomas.

Lee Ford[30] duplicated Shealy's work as closely as possible in 27 cats and observed no acute hemorrhage after exposing the epidural space to chymopapain. Necropsies done between 1 and 14 weeks after exposure of the dura to chymopapain showed no inflammatory changes or adhesions greater than those seen in control laminectomies. Two animals injected intrathecally died within 24 hours of extensive hemorrhage in the subarachnoid space. One animal survived such an injection. Ford could not demonstrate necrosis or hemorrhage of the liver or spleen as described by Shealy. Nor could he demonstrate aneurysms, severe inflammatory changes, arteritis, or arachnoiditis.

CLINICAL CORRELATION WITH LABORATORY FINDINGS

Twenty-nine percent (22 of 75) of Smith and Brown's patients had an epidural leakage of contrast dye at discography. Twenty-one of these had rapid relief of their sciatica. There was no difference in treatment outcome between the patients who had a leakage of dye at the time of discography and those who did not. Forty thousand patients later, numerous subsequent surgical observations have failed to show a deleterious effect of chymopapain in the epidural space of humans.

The problem of neural toxicity from chymopapain was not to be rationally studied until 1976, when Rydevik and associates[31] published their experimental model. They showed that chymopapain did not acutely block nerve conduction but did impair the blood-nerve barrier by damaging the intraneural microvessels, resulting in intraneural edema. The long-term consequences of this sequence were nerve tissue degeneration, intraneural fibrosis, and impaired nerve function.

Caution should be exercised in interpreting the adverse reactions of the initial group of patients treated with chymopapain. Most had had discograms performed with Hypaque. Anaphylaxis, as well as acute generalized seizures, are two of the toxic—sometimes fatal—side effects of this contrast agent.[32] When it is accidentally injected into the lumbar subarachnoid space, a generalized seizure may result, although seizures were not observed in the chemonucleolysis patients described in the literature. The extradural injection route and the use of Conray-60 in later clinical trials alleviated some of the potential problems associated with Hypaque.

Data from Stern[33] on the pharmacology of chymopapain helped to explain the immediate beneficial effects of intradiscal injection. An increase in chondroitin-6-sulfate in patients' urine within the first 24 hours after injection was interpreted as a reflection of chymopapain's enzymatic breakdown of the disc.

Stern had previously shown (1967)[34] that tissue residue decreased and nitrogen was released into the supernatant solution within 4 hours after exposing human nucleus pulposus to chymopapain in vitro. Small amounts of chymopapain catalyzed rapid reductions in the viscosity of the water-soluble portion of the nucleus pulposus within 1 hour after the chondromucoprotein was exposed to the enzyme. It was surmised that chymopapain causes an immediate degradation of chondromucoprotein and, therefore, a rapid reduction of intradiscal pressure.

Gesler[35] showed that chymopapain is bound rapidly, both in vitro and in vivo, to the acid mucopolysaccharide of the nucleus pulposus. At tissue pH, chymopapain has a positive charge, whereas the acid proteoglycans of the nucleus pulposus have a negative charge. Compared to papain, bacterial proteases, and trypsin, chymopapain was the most effective enzyme for dissolving the nucleus pulposus and had the least effect on the annulus fibrosus. The minimum effective dose of chymopapain to dissolve the nucleus pulposus in rabbits, cats, dogs and monkeys compared to the maximum tolerated dose administered epidurally or intradiscally, showed that the margin of safety was in the order of 300 to 1,000 times according to Gesler. However, there appears to be no margin of safety if the enzyme is injected directly into the subarachnoid space.

The high intrathecal toxicity is due to the fact that the pia-arachnoid membrane contains a dense microvascular network, which is readily exposed to intrathecally injected substances. Brånemark[36] and his associates showed quite elegantly that, whenever chymopapain comes into direct contact with microvasculature, it dissolves the proteoglycan-binding substance between endothelial cells, with subsequent rupture of the capillary and release of blood corpuscles. When a solution containing 5 mg of chymopapain per cc (0.5%) was placed on rabbit tibial nerves, the circulation in the microvasculature of the nerve was reduced immediately and numerous thromboemboli formed. Within minutes, micro-bleeding appeared. After 5 minutes, intrafascicular circulation was affected, and the changes persisted throughout the observation.

Angiography of the rabbit lumbar spine 3 months after intradiscal enzyme injection of a 1% solution demonstrated no evidence of abnormality of the microvasculature around the discs. The discs were narrowed, and the nucleus pulposus was gone. When a 0.1% solution of chymopapain was injected, there was no evidence of damage to the disc. However, 0.05 ml of a 0.3% enzyme solution completely dissolved the nucleus pulposus in all cases. The disc narrowing and dissolution of the nucleus pulposus were irreversible. There were no changes in the vascular pattern around the disc.

Whenever chymopapain came into direct contact with microcirculation, it caused an immediate and obvious dose-related rupture of the vessels. Chymopapain levels below 0.1% caused changes that were reversible; higher concentrations caused bleeding with permanent changes. These direct vital microscopic observations were dramatic demonstrations of the danger of injecting chymopapain into the subarachnoid space. All clinical trials were performed with 0.4% (4 mg/cc) solution of chymopapain.

REFERENCES

1. Hirsch C.: Studies on the pathology of low back pain. *J. Bone Joint Surg.* 41B:237, 1959.
2. Smith L., Garvin P.J., Jennings R.B.: Enzyme dissolution of the nucleus pulposus. *Nature* 198:1311, 1963.
3. Hirsch C., Schajowicz F.: Studies on structural changes in the lumbar annulus fibrosus. *Acta Orthop. Scand.* 22:184, 1952.
4. Mineiro J.D.: Coluna vertebral humana. Alguna aspectos da sua estruturae vascularizacao. Ph.D. thesis, University of Lisbon, 1965.

5. Jackson H.B., Winkelmann R.K., Bickel W.H.: Nerve endings in the human lumbar spinal column and related structures. *J. Bone Joint Surg.* 48A:1272, 1966.

6. Nachemson A., Morris J.M.: In vivo measurements of intradiscal pressure discometry: A method for the determination of pressure in the lower lumbar discs. *J. Bone Joint Surg.* 46A:1077, 1964.

7. Hirsch C.: Etiology and pathogenesis of low back pain. *Isr. J. Med. Sci.* 2:362, 1966.

8. Coventry M.B., Ghormley R.K., Kernohan J.W.: The intervertebral disc: Its microscopic anatomy and pathology. *J. Bone Joint Surg.* 27:105 (Part I), 233 (Part II), 460 (Part III), 1945.

9. Sylven B.: On the biology of nucleus pulposus. *Acta Orthop. Scand.* 20:275, 1950.

10. Brown M.D.: The Pathophysiology of the Intervertebral Disc. Ph.D. thesis, Thomas Jefferson University, Philadelphia, 1969.

11. Charnley J.: The imbibition of fluid as a cause of herniation of the nucleus pulposus. *Lancet,* p 124, Jan. 19, 1952.

12. Knutsson F.: The instability associated with disc degeneration in the lumbar spine. *Acta Radiol.* 25:593, 1944.

13. Bobechko W.P., Hirsch C.: Autoimmune response to nucleus pulposus in the rabbit. *J. Bone Joint Surg.* 47B:574, 1965.

14. Thomas L.: Reversible collapse of rabbits' ears after intravenous papain and prevention of recovery by cortisone. *J. Exp. Med.* 104:245, 1956.

15. McCluskey R.T., Thomas L.: Removal of cartilage matrix, in vivo, by papain. Identification of crystalline papain protease as cause of phenomenon. *J. Exp. Med.* 108:371, 1958.

16. Bryant J.H., Leder I.G., Stetlen D., Jr.: The release of chondroitin sulfate from rabbit cartilage following the intravenous injection of crude papain. *Arch. Biochem.* 76:122, 1958.

17. Ball E.J.: A new treatment of ganglion. *Am. J. Surg.* 50:722, 1940.

18. Feffer H.L.: Treatment of low back and sciatic pain by the injection of hydrocortisone into degenerated intervertebral discs. *J. Bone Joint Surg.* 38A:585, 1956.

19. Smith L.: Enzyme dissolution of nucleus pulposus in humans. *J.A.M.A.* 18:137, 1964.

20. Erlacher P.R.: Nucleography. *J. Bone Joint Surg.* 34B:204, 1952.

21. Saunders E.C.: Treatment of the canine intervertebral disc syndrome with chymopapain. *J. Am. Vet. Med. Assoc.* 145:893, 1964.

22. Smith L., Brown J.E.: Treatment of lumbar intervertebral disc lesions by direct injection of chymopapain. *J. Bone Joint Surg.* 49B:502, 1967.

23. Edholm P., Fernstrom I., Lindblom K.: Extradural lumbar disk puncture. *Acta Radiol.* [*Diagn.*] *(Stockh.)* 6:322, 1967.

24. Garvin P.J., Jennings R.B., Smith L., Gesler, R.M.: Chymopapain: A pharmacologic and toxicologic evaluation in experimental animals. *Clin. Orthop.* 41:204, 1965.

25. Howland W.J., Curry J.L.: Experimental studies of Pantopaque arachnoiditis. I. Animal studies. *Radiology* 37:253, 1966.

26. Shealy C.N.: Dangers of spinal injections without proper diagnosis. *J.A.M.A.* 197:156, 1966.

27. Holt E.P., Jr.: Fallacy of cervical discography. *J.A.M.A.* 188:799, 1964.

28. Shealy C.N.: Tissue reactions to chymopapain in cats. *J. Neurosurg.* 26:327, 1967.

29. MacNab I.: Personal communication, 1973.

30. Ford L.T.: Experimental study of chymopapain in cats. *Clin. Orthop.* 67:68, 1969.

31. Rydevik B., Brånemark P.I., Nordberg C., et al.: Effects of chymopapain on nerve tissue. *Spine* 1:137, 1976.

32. Wollin D.G., Lamon C.B., Cawley A.J., Wortzman G.: Neurotoxic effect of water-soluble contrast media in spinal canal with emphasis on appropriate management. *J. Can. Assoc. Radiol.* 18:296, 1967.

33. Stern I.J., Cosmas F., Smith L.: Urinary polyuronide excretion in man after enzymic dissolution of the chondromucous protein of the intervertebral disc or surgical stress. *Clin. Chim. Acta* 21:181, 1968.

34. Stern I.J., Smith L.: Dissolution by chymopapain in vitro of tissue from normal or prolapsed intervertebral disks. *Clin. Orthop.* 50:269, 1967.

35. Gesler R.M.: Pharmacologic properties of chymopapain. *Clin. Orthop.* 67:47, 1969.

36. Brånemark P.I., Ekholm R., Lundskog J., et al.: Tissue response to chymopapain in different concentrations: Animal investigations on microvascular effects. *Clin. Orthop.* 67:52, 1969.

2 / Clinical Trials With Chymopapain

PHASES OF NEW DRUG TRIALS

IN ORDER TO CLINICALLY TEST a new drug on humans in the United States, the manufacturer must obtain an investigational new drug number (IND) from the Food and Drug Administration (FDA).[1] Before this number is assigned, the pharmacology of the drug, its efficacy, toxicity, and margin of safety must be documented in animal studies.

Phase I, the first trial in man, establishes the nature, possible benefits, and risks of the drug. Its efficacy must then be proved in a controlled trial, Phase II. Once efficacy has been established, usually through a randomized double-blind study, the drug moves into Phase III trials, in which large numbers of patients are treated. The drug is still not available commercially in Phase III but is limited to investigators who make scientific observations, and file both initial and follow-up patient evaluations with the manufacturer and with the FDA. Finally, the drug is ready for Phase IV, when it becomes available commercially. However, physicians must still file reports of adverse reactions.

The development of chymopapain was peculiar in that, following Phase I (1963–1969) it went directly into Phase III trials because the original investigators thought that a controlled study was impossible, as well as unethical.[2] This is discussed more fully in Chapter 3.

PHASE I

The first-phase clinical trials (1963–1969) on chymopapain culminated in a symposium published in 1969.[3] In this symposium, Lyman Smith coined the term "chemonucleolysis,"[4] defining it as the treatment of intervertebral disc lesions by the intradiscal injection of the enzyme chymopapain. The term has now come to mean the treatment of intervertebral disc lesions by intradiscal injection of any lysing agent.[5]

Smith reported his experience with 150 patients who had been followed from 6 to 60 months. Only 30 had undergone previous myelography, but all had had discograms confirming the diagnosis. Thirty-five percent of the patients experienced severe lumbar back pain 12 to 36 hours after injection. The severity and duration of the pain had no relation to the outcome of the case, the disc injected, or the chymopapain dosage. Fifty-one patients had mild, recurring muscle spasms, and 13% had no complaints of back pain whatsoever after injection.

15

Seventy-three percent experienced relief from sciatica within the first 24 hours, which implies prompt decompression of the nerve root. The in vitro effect of chymopapain's diminishing the viscosity of chondromucoprotein and the rapid increase in urinary excretion of chondrotin-6-sulfate after intradiscal injection explain the prompt pain relief. However, permanent relief of leg pain from the intradiscal injection of hydrocortisone,[6] local anesthetic, or saline[7] has been reported by other authors.

The immediate relief of sciatica was not complete; total relief of pain required between 4 and 6 weeks following injection. Most patients with sedentary occupations returned to work within 3 weeks, while those with more strenuous jobs returned to work after more than 6 weeks.

Of those patients with no previous spinal surgery, 88.3% had good results, only 8.1% had poor results. Patients with previous spinal surgery had 68.8% good results, and 18.1%, poor results. Nine patients underwent laminectomy after chymopapain injection. The only consistent finding was the lack of deleterious effect from the chymopapain injections. Most of the 257 discs injected in the 150 patients narrowed within the first week. Five patients had recurrent disc protrusions 18 to 25 months after injection. Forty-four patients were examined for antibodies to chymopapain up to 2 years following injection; none were found.

Early in Phase I trials two major neurologic deficits, although adequately explained, prompted an 8-month moratorium on further injections in humans while further animal experiments were repeated and expanded to include primates.[8] Garvin et al. reported these pharmacologic and toxicologic evaluations.[9] The clinical trial resumed; and, by 1969, eight investigators had performed chemonucleolysis on approximately 600 patients. The eight investigators were Joseph Brown, Philip Day, Lee Ford, Ian MacNab, George Schoedinger, Lyman Smith, W. J. Stewart, and Dennis Weiner.

Lee Ford's experience[10] with 126 patients was similar to that of Smith and Brown (Table 2–1). One of his patients developed immediate anaphylactic shock and was later found to be allergic to Adolph's meat tenderizer, which contains papain. The chymopapain caused a precipitous fall in blood pressure to 45 mm Hg, and it remained low for an hour

TABLE 2–1.—RESULTS OF CLINICAL TRIALS OF
CHYMOPAPAIN, 1963–1969

| INVESTIGATOR | NO. OF PATIENTS | RESULTS | | |
		Good	Fair	Poor
L. Smith[4]	150	125	11	14
P. Day[12]	135	105	23	7
L. Ford[10]	126	74	28	24
W. Stewart[11]	40	28	8	4
Total	451	332 (73%)	70 (16%)	49 (11%)

despite resuscitative measures. She was treated with large doses of intravenous steroids and recovered after 48 hours, eventually to have good treatment results.

Ford also treated two patients with thoracic discs, one at T-9 and one at T-11. Both had a satisfactory outcome. This is the only reference in the literature to treatment of thoracic discs by chemonucleolysis.

Stewart[11] reported on 40 patients ranging in age from 20 to 73 and found no relationship between the number of discs injected and the end results. He had difficulty penetrating the L-5–S-1 disc space of one patient and abandoned the procedure.

Day[12] preceded his injections by discograms with Renografin, using the lateral approach. Of 135 patients, three suffered anaphylactic reactions. Only one patient had an antibody to chymopapain in the postinjection phase, and Day surmised that the patients were allergic to Renografin. He stated that, "in clear-cut cases" (see Table 1–1), 95% of the patients had an excellent or good response, whereas in a "less desirable group of patients" there was only a 60% chance of an excellent or good result. Seven patients of the 135 treated were unimproved.

Brown,[13] redescribing his earlier experience with 23 patients treated by chemonucleolysis, concluded that neither the symptoms, the physical findings, the presence of compensation or litigation, the number of discs injected, nor the amount of postinjection disc space narrowing had any influence over the end results.

In the same symposium, Henry Feffer[14] reported the results of therapeutic intradiscal hydrocortisone injections. He noted long-term remission of symptoms in 46.7% of 244 patients treated. He found that patients in whom back symptoms predominated responded more favorably than those patients who suffered primarily from sciatica or radiculopathy. Also, the patients who responded were more apt to be over age 50. These results are interesting when compared to subsequent careful studies by Wiltse[15] that demonstrated intradiscal chymopapain injection is more effective in younger patients with predominantly leg-pain complaints.

PHASE III

Between 1969 and 1975, chymopapain was tested in more than 16,000 patients. Between 1974 and 1975, a Phase II controlled double-blind study comparing chymopapain to placebo was performed (Table 2–2). After 1975, the investigational new drug number was withdrawn from FDA by Baxter Travenol Laboratories because of failure to demonstrate efficacy in this trial.[16] However, chymopapain became commercially available outside the United States (Phase IV). In the United States and Australia, further controlled studies were performed.

Table 2–2.—Chymopapain And Collagenase: Brief Chronology of
Clinical Trials

DATE		INVESTIGATOR	TOPIC
Chymopapain			
1959		Hirsch	Concept of enzymatic injection treatment
1963 ⎫		Smith	Efficacy and toxicity in animals
1964 ⎭		Smith	Results in 10 patients
	Phase I		
1969 ⎫			
	Phase III	Wiltse et al.	
1974 ⎭			
	Phase II		Double-blind study
1975 ⎫			
	Phase IV		Canada
1982 ⎭			
	Phase II		U.S.A. and Australia
Collagenase			
1958		Mandl	Purified *C. histolyticum* collagenase
1968		Sussman	Discolysis with collagenase in vitro
1979		Bromley	Efficacy and toxicity collagenase in animals
March ⎤		Bromley	82 patients
	Phase I	Gomez	
		Sussman	
1980 ⎟			
June ⎦			
	Phase II	Bromley	Double-blind study, 30 patients
1981 ⎫			
November ⎬			
1982 ⎫			
April ⎭		Bromley	
	Phase III	Gomez	
		Brown et al.	

Organization of the literature as shown in Table 2–2 makes it easier
to understand why chymopapain was not released until 1982. Bizarre as
it may seem in retrospect, between 1979 and 1982 an alternative enzyme—collagenase—passed through a Phase I clinical trial into Phase
II and was proved efficacious in as few as 30 selected patients in a well-
designed double-blind protocol comparing collagenase to saline.[17] The
collagenase trial passed into Phase III in January 1982, before the
Phase II approval of chymopapain.

Between 1969 and 1975, several more investigators published on che-
monucleolysis with chymopapain: Mark Brown, Robert Daroff, Edmond
Graham, Brian Huncke, Gerald Jabbaay, George Lucas, John Mc-
Culloch, Eugene Nordby, Burton Onofrio, Robert Sullivan, and Leon
Wiltse.

Between 1969 and 1975, the number of U.S. investigators increased
from eight to 55 orthopedists and neurosurgeons. Approximately 600
patients were treated in 1969, increasing to almost 17,000 by the end of

1975. This number included approximately 300 patients from continental Europe, England, Australia, Sweden, and Canada.

Clinical Data

MacNab and associates[18] published an outstanding clinical investigation in 1971. In additional toxicology studies, they determined that rabbits and dogs tolerated intradiscal and epidural doses of chymopapain 1,000 times greater than the dose required to dissolve the nucleus pulposus.

They also pointed out that Hypaque, the contrast dye utilized then, was extremely toxic to rabbits, dogs, and cats when injected intrathecally in doses as small as 0.2 mg per kilogram.

They initially thought that chymopapain functioned by rapidly inducing narrowing and stiffening of the unstable degenerated intervertebral disc—a concept similar to a theory of Carl Hirsch. On this basis, they gave 33 patients intradiscal injections of chymopapain during two- and three-level spinal fusions. One patient developed pseudoarthrosis. No definitive conclusions could be gleaned from this technique, and the concept was abandoned.

MacNab et al. then treated 100 patients with degenerative disease of the motion segment unit—making the important distinction between the patient with spinal stenosis or herniated disc and the patient with pure back pain without leg pain. They were the first to report performing the procedure under local anesthesia to avoid penetrating a nerve root. One-third of the patients had relief of leg pain before leaving the x-ray department. None of the patients were made worse by the procedure.

To analyze their results, MacNab et al. separated from their original 100 patients a group of 54 "simple" disc patients who had not responded to 6 weeks of bedrest and were ideal candidates for surgery. The patients all had objective evidence of nerve root involvement. Of these 54 patients, 85% obtained complete relief of their symptoms. Follow-up was 6 to 18 months for this group. Only 25% of the patients with back pain alone or spinal stenosis had satisfactory relief of symptoms. Patients with complicating factors such as obesity, diabetes, and gross emotional overlay had a successful outcome 64% of the time. In 10 patients, Pantopaque was left in the subarachnoid space, and new x-rays were taken at various intervals after chemonucleolysis. The patients showed no evidence of change in the myelographic defect.

It is interesting to note that, of the 100 patients injected, one had an immediate anaphylactic reaction with a drop in blood pressure and urticaria, and a second patient had a delayed sensitivity reaction with skin rash 10 days after injection. It was becoming apparent that chymopapain was associated with a relatively high number of systemic allergic reactions.

CHEMONUCLEOLYSIS VERSUS SURGERY

Nordby and Lucas[19] compared results in 100 consecutive patients treated by laminectomy and disc excision to results in 100 patients injected with chymopapain. Surgery produced acceptable results in 68%, compared with 90% acceptable results with chemonucleolysis. There were fewer patients in the "poor" category with chemonucleolysis, and none of the patients were made worse by the treatment. Chemonucleolysis patients averaged 9 days of hospitalization, compared with 12 days for the laminectomy patients. The chemonucleolysis patients returned to work 66 days (on the average) following treatment, compared with 202 days following laminectomy. Nordby and Lucas concluded that 75% of laminectomies could be avoided by the use of chemonucleolysis.

A LARGE CLINICAL TRIAL

The classic experience with the use of chemonucleolysis in 1,200 patients with lumbar disc disease was reported by Leon Wiltse[20] following a prospective protocol performed by 18 orthopedists and neurosurgeons between 1968 and 1975. They reported in detail their experience with 500 patients who had at least a 3-year follow-up.

Wiltse's study made important contributions to our knowledge of the effects of chymopapain on epidural tissue, appropriate dyes in discography, surgery after chemonucleolysis, chemonucleolysis and neurologic deficits, and sensitivity reactions to chymopapain.

Effects of Chymopapain on Epidural Tissue

In 25% of Wiltse's patients, x-ray contrast dye had leaked into the epidural space during discography. In three of these patients, subsequent laminectomy and biopsy of tissue from the epidural space revealed no changes attributable to chymopapain.

Appropriate Discogram Dye

In the course of his study, Wiltse compared the intrathecal toxicity of Hypaque to Conray-60 (iothalmate meglumine). Hypaque was found to be 50 to 100 times more toxic than Conray-60 when injected intrathecally. For this reason, he recommended Conray-60 for discograms.

Surgery After Failed Chemonucleolysis

In patients who had had no previous back surgery, 80% had satisfactory symptomatic relief with chemonucleolysis. Of the first 500 patients, 112 failed to obtain relief, and 56 of these required surgery. Of the patients who underwent surgery after failed chemonucleolysis, 74% had a satisfactory outcome.

The most common reason for failure of chemonucleolysis was a hard bulging annulus fibrosus combined with disc space narrowing which resulted in nerve root pressure. Five patients had spinal stenosis, four had disc herniations at a level other than the one injected, and five patients showed no change in the disc that would imply a previous injection.

Effects of Chemonucleolysis on Neurologic Deficits

Of the patients with neurologic deficit, 61% had reversal of reflex changes to normal, 83% had motor changes reverse to normal, and 77% of those with sensory deficits had reverse to normal. These changes were noted 1 year after injection and the figures confirmed by a comparative series of chemonucleolysis with chymopapain in 1980.[21] When compared to a one-year follow-up of surgery[22] for proved disc displacement, chemonucleolysis emerges as the gentler method of decompressing nerve roots with a more favorable response (Table 2–3).

Wiltse's group noted that approximately 50% of the patients had obtained optimal results by 4 months following injection, 75% by 6 months, and the remaining patients had plateaued by a year after injection. These investigators were impressed that the good results were not compromised by any findings of extruded discs. Nor did they find any correlation between disc narrowing of more than 5 mm after chemonucleolysis with a successful outcome of the procedure.

Sensitivity Reactions

Of Wiltse's total sample of 1,200 patients, 3% exhibited allergic reactions: nine patients (0.7%) had an immediate systemic anaphylactic reaction, 15 had an immediate mild systemic cutaneous reaction, and 11 had delayed cutaneous reactions in the form of hives. The second 600 patients in the series were pretreated with hydrocortisone and diphenhydramine (Benadryl). Only two patients developed anaphylaxis, one severe and one mild. Among the first 600 patients, none of whom were

TABLE 2–3.—REVERSAL OF
NEUROLOGIC DEFICIT TO NORMAL
FOLLOWING CHEMONUCLEOLYSIS
WITH CHYMOPAPAIN (%)

	CHYMOPAPAIN*	SURGERY[22]
Reflex	61	14
Motor	83	71
Sensory	71	33

*Average % from Wiltse's series, 1975[20] and Javid's[21] series, 1980.

pretreated with the steroid and antihistamine, seven had anaphylaxis. It was Wiltse's impression that both the incidence of anaphylaxis and the severity of the reaction were diminished by prophylactic treatment with hydrocortisone and diphenhydramine.

FAILURES OF CHEMONUCLEOLYSIS

Lyman Smith[23] reported three cases of immediate anaphylactic response to the first injection and one of anaphylaxis following a second injection of chymopapain. Ten additional patients had delayed allergic reactions, 11 had thrombophlebitis, and four had pulmonary emboli. One patient had a mild disc space infection.

Smith was the first to report that some patients, when followed with serial x-rays after intradiscal chymopapain injection, showed widening of the disc space after the initial narrowing. This was subsequently confirmed by Wiltse and his group. Smith had a 93% good or excellent response in the last 100 injections that he had performed because he became very strict in his criteria for selection of patients for the procedure.

HALF-LIFE OF CHYMOPAPAIN

Several advancements in the understanding of chemonucleolysis with chymopapain occurred between 1969 and 1975. One excellent article[24] showed that the α_2-macroglobulin serum component inhibited the action of chymopapain.

Seven patients undergoing chemonucleolysis with 4–20 mg of enzyme were monitored up to 1 week for plasma chymopapain immunologically reactive fragments (CIP). After 24 hours, initial plasma levels as high as 470 mg per milliliter had declined rapidly but were still detectable after 7 days. Small amounts of CIP were found in the urine of these patients. It was surmised that the low concentration and the inhibition by the α_2-macroglobulins of the CIP in the serum prevented proteolytic activity from this material outside the disc.

The amount of CIP in the serum varied greatly among patients. On cinefluoroscopy discography, we have seen a great deal of variation in the rapidity with which injected contrast dye leaves the disc. In approximately 15% of discs, contrast dye enters vascular channels instantaneously following injection. In our opinion, some failures of chemonucleolysis can be explained by this rapid loss of chondrolytic agent on intradiscal injection, giving the chymopapain insufficient time to bind to the substrate in the disc matrix. However, even if a total of 30 mg of chymopapain were to be directly injected intravascularly in humans, we do not think there would be untoward effects from the rapid dilution of the drug and inactivation by the α_2-macroglobulins.

PSYCHOGENIC FACTORS

A beautifully performed study concerning the relationships of psychometric evaluations to treatment outcome was published by Wiltse and Rocchio[25] in 1975. They showed that 57 patients with one to five preinjection objective neurologic deficits and the low average score of 64 on the hysteria and the hypochondriasis scales of the Minnesota Multiphasic Personality Inventory had an 87% chance of good or excellent results from chemonucleolysis with chymopapain. Forty-two patients had scores of 75 and over on the hysteria and hypochondriasis scales and the same number of objective preinjection organic findings as the first group, and they had only a 25% incidence of a good or excellent outcome. This study has important ramifications with respect to patient selection, particularly since the percentage of good and excellent results in the hysteria-hypochondriasis group was less than that for placebo care in subsequent controlled studies.

PHARMACOLOGY OF CHYMOPAPAIN

In a review of the pharmacology of chymopapain, Clark Watts and associates[26] emphasized the importance of clinical awareness of patients' low tolerance for intrathecally injected chymopapain. The exact margin of safety between effective and toxic doses in humans cannot be predicted on the basis of animal studies. In humans, the minimum effective dose for dissolving nucleus pulposus by intradiscal injection was estimated at between 2 and 4 mg per disc. Extrapolating from animal studies, the maximum tolerated intradiscal dose in man would approach 600 mg, leaving a margin of safety 150 times the effect of intradiscal dose.

NEUROTOXICITY

An elegant study of the effect of chymopapain on rabbit tibial nerves was published by Rydevik et al. in 1976.[27] They demonstrated that chymopapain had no *acute* effect on the electrical function of the nerves or axonal transport of proteins but did almost immediately impair the blood-nerve barrier of the intraneural microvessels, causing intrafascicular edema. The long-term consequences of these changes were degeneration of nerve fibers, intraneural fibrosis, an increase in the threshold of action potentials, and a delay in nerve conduction velocity. We think the clinical relevance of this study is that inadvertent exposure or spearing of the nerve root under general anesthesia during injection could lead to permanent nerve damage from chymopapain's action on the microvessels of the nerves.[28] On the basis of Rydevik's findings, we think that chymopapain has a potential for neural toxicity. But these findings should be kept in perspective with the results in more than 14,000 patients who had been treated with chymopapain at that time. These patients showed no increased nerve damage. On the contrary, their reversal rate of neurologic deficit to normal was higher after injection than after surgical decompression of lumbar nerve roots for disc disease.

ACTION OF CHYMOPAPAIN ON NUCLEUS PULPOSUS

Biochemical changes were noted in the nucleus pulposus removed at laminectomy following failure of relief from chemonucleolysis.[29] Six of the nine patients treated with chymopapain had reduced hexosamine in the disc material removed at surgery. This was further evidence that chymopapain did indeed reduce the proteoglycans of the nucleus pulposus when injected in vivo.

MORE CRITICISM OF CHYMOPAPAIN

In 1975, at the completion of the Phase III studies on chymopapain, Bernard Sussman[30] criticized the use of the enzyme. The intent of Sussman's article was obscured by the fact that he was a strong proponent of collagenase, which he had studied since 1967. His most valid criticism of the chymopapain trials was that "patients with herniated intervertebral discs undergo clinical remission during the first 2 months after onset of symptoms and that at any point in the subsequent course of this disease 50% of patients are in clinical remission." He thought that "any new intradiscal method should also be required to better the 47% improvement rate obtained safely by Feffer with intradiscal cortisone." Otherwise, the article reviewed previously known complications that had occurred in the clinical trials of over 8,000 patients.

SUMMARY OF COMPLICATIONS

In 1977, Clark Watts published a synopsis of all the complications from chemonucleolysis with chymopapain that had been observed in the first 13,700 patients treated.[31] There were a total of 401 complications, adverse reactions, and delayed untoward events, including eight deaths. Sensitivity reactions occurred in 1.5% of the total sample, neurologic complications in 0.4%, cardiovascular complications in 0.3%, and miscellaneous complications in 0.8%.

Sensitivity Reactions

Two hundred and seven patients had sensitivity reactions; of these, 77 had delayed reactions with cutaneous manifestations (itching and/or hives), which occurred 10 days to 3 weeks after injection.

One hundred and thirty patients had immediate systemic reactions, 53 of which were mild in nature, with hives, wheezing, and transient hypotension. Fifty-two patients had a moderately severe reaction that required supportive treatment measures. Twenty-five patients (0.2% of 13,700) had a severe anaphylactic reaction that required intensive care. Two of these patients died from this reaction. With only a 0.2% severe systemic allergic reaction rate, it is difficult to compile meaningful statistics on amelioration or prevention by pretreatment with hydrocortisone and diphenhydramine, as suggested by Wiltse and his associates.

Neurologic Complications

Forty-nine patients suffered neurologic complications, 19 of whom had transient temporary urinary retention. It is difficult to decide what caused this complication because some patients go into urinary retention from pain, bedrest, and/or narcotics. Nine patients had foot drop, and three had causalgia, which Watts interpreted as being secondary to needle penetration of nerves. Some of these complications might have been avoided by the use of local anesthesia for the injection.

Cardiovascular Complications

Thirty-four patients had cardiovascular reactions—15 with thrombophlebitis, 13 with pulmonary embolus, 2 with cardiac arrests, 2 with ruptured aortic aneurysms, and 2 with myocardial infarctions. One patient, a physician whom I treated during this period, developed a pulmonary embolus while on the x-ray table just prior to chemonucleolysis. The patient complained of pleuritic pain, which we interpreted as being caused by his position on the x-ray table. He had been bedridden with severe sciatica and cardiac arrhythmia for at least 10 days previously. This was a complication of conservative treatment of severe sciatica.

The majority of such complications can be prevented. Ten years ago, we were apt to prescribe strict bedrest for sciatica. Today, we hardly ever do, for fear of thromboembolic complications. The cardiovascular complications were not peculiar to chemonucleolysis but to the differential diagnosis and treatment of disc disease.

The ruptured aortic aneurysms were complications of misdiagnosis or coincidental disease. One occurred 3 months after injection of chymopapain. Cardiac arrest and myocardial infarctions are complications that can occur under any stressful circumstance.

TABLE 2–4.—Chymopapain Therapy and Surgery:
Comparison of Risks (%)

	COMPLICATIONS	MORTALITY	RECURRENT DISC
Chymopapain	3	0.03	1
Surgery	6	0.17	6

From Brown M.D.[34]

Miscellaneous Complications

A number of transient conditions such as ileitis, cystitis, psychosis, nonspecific headaches, nausea, vomiting, and adverse reactions to placebo can be seen in any stressful treatment regimen.[32] Twenty-two patients had discitis, a known complication of discography.[33]

Fatalities Following Chemonucleolysis

Of the eight deaths, two can be directly attributed to treatment with chymopapain. These were the result of anaphylactic reactions. One patient developed a disc space infection and chronic protracted septicemia, and died from subacute bacterial endocarditis 55 days later. This complication could have occurred with any intradiscal injection.

SAFETY COMPARED TO SURGERY

On comparing the nature, benefit, and risks of chemonucleolysis to large series of surgical disc excisions, it is my opinion that enzyme injection is at least five times safer than surgery (Table 2–4).[34]

REFERENCES

1. U.S. Food and Drug Administration: Federal Food, Drug, and Cosmetic Act, Section 505(i); Code of Federal Regulation, Title 21, Section 312.
2. Smith L., Brown J.E.: Treatment of lumbar intervertebral disc lesions by direct injection of chymopapain. *J. Bone Joint Surg.* 49-B:502, 1967.
3. Massie W. (ed.): Symposium on chemonucleolysis. *Clin. Orthop.* 67:2, 1969.
4. Smith L.: Chemonucleolysis. *Clin. Orthop.* 67:72, 1969.
5. American Academy of Orthopaedic Surgeons: *A Glossary on Spinal Terminology.* (Document 675–80.) Chicago, American Academy of Orthopaedic Surgeons, 1980.
6. Feffer H.L.: Treatment of low back and sciatic pain by the injection of hydrocortisone into degenerated intervertebral discs. *J. Bone Joint Surg.* 38A:585, 1956.
7. Hirsch C.: An attempt to diagnose the level of a disc lesion clinically by disc puncture. *Acta Orthop. Scand.* 19:132, 1948.
8. Smith L.: Chemonucleolysis. *Clin. Orthop.* 67:72, 1969.
9. Garvin P.J., Jennings R.B., Smith L., Gesler R.M.: Chymopapain: A pharmacologic and toxicologic evaluation in experimental animals. *Clin. Orthop.* 41:204, 1965.

10. Ford L.: Clinical use of chymopapain in lumbar and dorsal disk lesions: An end-result study. *Clin. Orthop.* 67:81, 1969.
11. Stewart W.J.: Lateral discograms and chemonucleolysis in the treatment of ruptured or deteriorated lumbar discs. *Clin. Orthop.* 67:88, 1969.
12. Day P.L.: Lateral approach for lumbar diskogram and chemonucleolysis. *Clin. Orthop.* 67:90, 1969.
13. Brown J.E.: Clinical studies on chemonucleolysis. *Clin. Orthop.* 67:94, 1969.
14. Feffer H.L.: Therapeutic intradiscal hydrocortisone: A long-term study. *Clin. Orthop.* 67:100, 1969.
15. Wiltse L.: Chemonucleolysis in ideal candidates for laminectomy. *The Spectator,* June 30, 1978.
16. Chymopapain pulled off IND status. *Med. World News* 16:38, Sept. 8, 1975.
17. Bromley J., Santaro A., Cohen P., et al.: Double blind evaluation of collagenase injection for herniated lumbar discs. Submitted for publication, 1982.
18. MacNab I., McCullouch J.A., Winer D.S., et al.: Chemonucleolysis. *Can. J. Surg.* 14:280, 1971.
19. Nordby E.J., Lucas G.L.: A comparative analysis of lumbar disc disease treated by laminectomy or chemonucleolysis. *Clin. Orthop.* 90:119, 1973.
20. Wiltse L.L.: Chymopapain chemonucleolysis in lumbar disk disease. *J.A.M.A.* 233:1164, 1975.
21. Javid M.: Treatment of herniated lumbar disc syndrome with chymopapain. *J.A.M.A.* 243:2043, 1980.
22. Knutsson B.: How often do the neurological signs disappear after the operation of a herniated disc? *Acta Orthop. Scand.* 32:352, 1962.
23. Smith L.: Failures with chemonucleolysis. *Orthop. Clin. North Am.* 1:255, 1975.
24. Kapsalis A.A., Stern I.J., Bernstein I.: The fate of chymopapain injected for therapy in intervertebral disk disease. *J. Lab. Clin. Med.* 83:532, 1974.
25. Wiltse L.L., Rocchio P.D.: Preoperative psychological tests as predictors of success of chemonucleolysis in the treatment of the low back syndrome. *J. Bone Joint Surg.* 57A:478, 1975.
26. Watts C., Knighton R., Roulhac G.: Chymopapain treatment of intervertebral disc disease. *J. Neurosurg.* 42:374, 1975.
27. Rydevik B., Brånemark P.I., Nordberg C., et al.: Effects of chymopapain on nerve tissue. *Spine* 1:137, 1976.
28. Nordby E.J., Brown M.D.: Present status of chymopapain and chemonucleolysis. *Clin. Orthop.* 129:79, 1977.
29. Zaleske D.J., Ehrlich M.G., Huddleston J.I, Jr.: Combined biochemical and clinical investigation of chemonucleolysis failures. *Clin. Orthop.* 126:121, 1977.
30. Sussman B.J.: Inadequacies and hazards of chymopapain injections as treatment for intervertebral disc disease. *J. Neurosurg.* 42:389, 1975.
31. Watts C.: Complications of chemonucleolysis for lumbar disc disease. *Neurosurgery* 1:2, 1977.
32. Beecher H.K.: Powerful placebo. *J.A.M.A.* 159:1602, 1955.
33. Collis J.S., Jr.: *Lumbar Discography.* Springfield, Ill., Charles C Thomas, Publisher, 1963.
34. Brown M.D.: Chemonucleolysis with Discase: Technique, results, case reports. *Spine* 1:115, 1976; Erratum, 1:161, 1976.

3 / Controlled Studies in the Treatment of Disc Disease

BY THE END OF 1974, more than 15,000 patients with disc disease had been injected with chymopapain, and a decision concerning its commercial release was to be made by the Food and Drug Administration (FDA) at the request of Baxter Travenol Laboratories.

Based on information from the clinical trials, the benefit and risk ratio of the drug seemed appropriate for its intradiscal usage. J. Richard Crout, Director of the FDA Bureau of Drugs issued a statement: "We are presently working out the details of labeling and the mechanism of Phase IV studies and marketing procedures."[1] Margaret A. Clark, Acting Director, Division of Surgical and Dental Drug Products, also stated that the FDA intended to approve chymopapain (Discase) for Phase IV studies.[2] Clark had invited comments from all interested persons prior to the FDA's published notice. In the same publication, the American Association of Neurologic Surgeons recommended further clinical studies of the drug in the form of double-blind trials in medical centers under the direction of neurologic surgeons.[3] They also recommended further investigation under a Phase III protocol.

CHYMOPAPAIN: PHASE II (1974–1975)

Prior to 1974, the original investigators of chymopapain had considered a controlled double-blind study unethical. They cited the Declaration of Helsinki guidelines for clinical research as support for their position. One of the recommendations in the declaration reads: "Clinical research cannot legitimately be carried out unless the importance of the objective is in proportion to the inherent risk to the subject."[4] Approximately 15,000 patients had been treated by chemonucleolysis, and a workshop sponsored by the American Academy of Orthopaedic Surgeons reported that 72% of 6,752 patients experienced satisfactory symptomatic relief following intradiscal injection of Discase.[5] Some clinical researchers thought that the spontaneous cure rate for disc herniation was somewhere between 40% and 70% of patients.[6] To expose a large number of patients to a treatment with a 1% risk of systemic sensitivity reaction without proved efficacy greater than the spontaneous cure rate was thought to be unethical by several investigators.[7]

Henry K. Beecher[8] stated the case quite succinctly: "A valid design of surgical activity is most important when the principal change to be produced by a surgical procedure is subjective." A controlled study on the effect of internal mammary artery ligation showed that a surgical procedure for a painful condition can exert a powerful placebo effect that can result in improvement of subjective complaints as well as objective findings.[9] The decision by physicians to treat low back pain and sciatica by chemonucleolysis with chymopapain was a situation very similar to that faced by surgeons who were being told that anginal pain was dramatically relieved by internal mammary artery ligation. The blinded surgical trial eliminated this procedure immediately. No one could argue that the risk of an unnecessary discogram and intradiscal placebo injection to determine the efficacy of chymopapain was less serious than a surgical exposure without ligation (placebo) of the internal mammary artery.[10]

STUDY DESIGN

Robert Aussman, Medical Director of Travenol Laboratories, enlisted four medical centers (University of Miami School of Medicine; University of Minnesota School of Medicine; Walter Reed Army Medical Center; and Veterans Administration Hospital, San Francisco) to perform a double-blind study comparing Discase (Travenol's preparation of chymopapain) to a placebo in patients with proved lumbar disc displacement.[11] Only the "active" ingredient in Discase was deleted to make up the placebo. Therefore, the placebo contained 20 mg sodium iothalamate, 3.5 mg cysteine hydrochloride, and 0.3 mg disodium edetate (EDTA). Cysteine hydrochloride monohydrate and EDTA are activators of chymopapain and are present in Discase. Sodium iothalamate was added so that the lyophilized unreconstituted placebo appeared identical in the vial to unreconstituted Discase. The addition of 20 mg of this dye to the placebo was considered inconsequential, since all injections were preceded by a discogram with the same contrast.

Coded vials of the lyophilized Discase or placebo in a prerandomized sequence were supplied to each investigating team. One vial was selected for each patient and reconstituted with 5 ml of sterile water for injection, and 1 ml of the dissolved drug was injected through a one-way Milex filter. All patients were injected under local anesthesia with anesthesia standby. They had been pretreated with diphenhydramine and hydrocortisone, and a discogram with 60% sodium iothalamate was performed 15 minutes before a coded vial's contents were injected.[11]

Measurement of Outcome

Three measures to determine results were utilized: the code break rate, the physician evaluation data sheet, and two telephone polls. The first poll, of 54 patients, was conducted by Price Waterhouse[12] in June 1975; the second poll was performed by Rabin Research Institute[13] in October 1975 on 94 patients, utilizing a modified questionnaire. Data were collected and statistics analyzed by the Departments of Clinical Research and Regulatory Affairs in the biostatistical service of Travenol Laboratories.[14]

Results

No matter how these results were analyzed (code break, patients' or doctors' perception of outcome, independent analysis by orthopedist Fred Reynolds[15] or neurosurgeon Robert Knighton,[16] or a 4-year follow-up of patients who underwent surgery[17]), there was no significant difference between those patients who received Discase and those who received placebo.

Analysis of Results

There were 3 publications of the original double-blind study[18, 19, 20] results of chemonucleolysis. In one of these,[19] we criticized the design of the study for 3 reasons.

First, we thought that the code break came too early. Before 6 weeks had elapsed (6 weeks being the optimum time interval after injection for relief from chemonucleolysis), 65% of patients who received Discase had broken code, versus 57% of patients who received placebo. After six weeks, the rate of code break for Discase patients was 40%, versus 50% for placebo patients. Since Discase causes reactive change in the intervertebral joint secondary to disc space narrowing, we knew that Discase could temporarily increase pain and thus encourage an unnecessarily early code break.

Second, the arbitrarily determined fixed dose of Discase was insufficient. The American Academy of Orthopaedic Surgeons' Committee on Chymopapain[5] had previously reported that a patient's clinical improvement was related to the amount of injected Discase (Table 3–1). Patients receiving 1 ml of Discase (containing 4 mg, or 2,000 units, of chymopapain) per disc had a higher failure rate than those who received larger amounts per disc. The initial double-blind study fixed the dose at 1 ml per disc despite the committee's report and the fact that the amount of agent accepted by the discs varied between 2 and 4 ml before the test injection. We thought that the prescribed amount of Discase was insufficient to achieve maximum therapeutic efficacy and thus biased the study results.

Finally, we thought that the placebo was not inert and may have had some therapeutic effect. The Walter Reed Army Medical Center double-blind evaluation reports 86% relief of leg pain with placebo and 71% with Discase within 24 hours after the injection.[18] We thought that ei-

TABLE 3–1.—Effects of Discase Dosage on
Clinical Improvement

DOSE PER DISC (MG)	NO. PATIENTS	IMPROVEMENT (%)		
		Marked	Slight	None
1–4	210	63.2	16.5	20.3
4–6	5,495	71.5	14.1	15.8
>6	1,295	72.0	14.0	14.0

From American Academy of Orthopaedic Surgeons.[5]

ther the cysteine hydrochloride and/or the EDTA in both the Discase and the placebo had some temporary analgesic effect that confused the overall outcome of the study.[19]

Based on the three factors of early code break, dose limitation, and lack of true placebo control, we recommended a repeat study with better design to eliminate code breaks until 6 weeks had elapsed after injection, to permit discretion in determining the amount of Discase injected (making it equivalent to the amount of discogram dye injected), and to utilize a true placebo, such as saline. We recommended that the study compare Discase to CEI, the placebo in the original study, to saline in a triple-blind study.[19, 21]

Long-Term Follow-Up

Martins and associates[20] reported the late results of double-blind evaluations of chemonucleolysis in 1978. One year or more after injection, 55% of those treated with chymopapain and 46% of those treated with placebo had satisfactory symptomatic relief. In a subset of 45 patients— 18 who received Discase, 27 who received placebo, and all of whom had objective evidence of radiculopathy before injection—67% of the enzyme-treated patients were successful, compared with 48% of the placebo-treated patients (Table 3–2). They stated, "To discard chemonucleolysis on the basis of this one small clinical trial may be premature," and they recommended further studies.

In the 4-year follow-up telephone survey at the University of Miami School of Medicine,[17] of 61 patients who participated in the original double-blind study, we found that (45%) of those who received Discase required surgery, versus 50% of those that received placebo (CEI) (Table 3–3). Taking into account the number of injections rather than the number of patients (six patients received a combination of two injections—failed placebo, then Discase), 46% of the Discase patients required surgery, versus 58% of the CEI patients. It is interesting that the average time interval between injection and surgery was 5.3 months for the placebo patients, versus 15.1 months for the Discase-injected patients. These intervals were calculated for patients who received one

TABLE 3–2.—PERCENTAGE OF SATISFACTORY OUTCOME (NO CODE BREAK) IN VARIOUS PROSPECTIVE DOUBLE-BLIND STUDIES OF CHEMONUCLEOLYSIS DRUGS

DATE, STUDY, REFERENCE	NO. PATIENTS	DISCASE	COLLAGENASE	CEI	SALINE
1975—double-blind[19]	104	59		50	—
1981—triple-blind[26]	120	78		57	22
1982—Australian double-blind[27]	60	80		—	57
1981—double-blind[32]	30		86		33

TABLE 3–3.—PATIENTS* SUBSEQUENTLY REQUIRING SURGERY

CHEMONUCLEOLYSIS AGENT	SURGERY	NO SURGERY
Discase	13 (45%)	16
Placebo (CEI)	16 (50%)	16

*From original double-blind study.[17]

injection only. We interpreted these results to mean that the Discase-treated patients had a temporary beneficial result from an insufficient amount of enzyme. Therefore, it took three times as long for failure to occur to the point that surgery was required following the Discase injection, as compared with the CEI injection.

FURTHER CONTROLLED STUDIES OF DISC DISEASE (1975–1982)

A comparison of the original double-blind study to a subsequent randomized study of disc displacement treatment by conservative versus operative care will throw some light on the factors of patient selection and expected outcome from conservative care or treatment with placebos.

Henrik Weber[22, 23] published the results of 14 days of strict bedrest and conservative care in 280 consecutive patients with diagnosed herniated disc. Sixty-seven patients had definite indications for surgery and were operated on. Eighty-seven patients had improved to the point where no further care was required. In the 126 remaining patients between the ages of 25 and 55, the symptoms and/or signs of disc disease still warranted further treatment. There was a relative indication for surgery in this group, and these patients were randomized into two subgroups. Patients in one subgroup continued on conservative care; patients in the other subgroup were operated on. At 4 years follow-up, 67% of the conservatively treated patients had a satisfactory outcome. Eighty-six percent of the surgically treated patients had satisfactory results. Although Weber's statisticians did not think it necessary to include 17 patients in the conservatively treated group who subsequently underwent surgery as failed results for the conservative group, we did. Therefore, we calculated a 33% incidence of unsatisfactory results in the conservatively treated group, versus a 14% unsatisfactory outcome in the surgically treated group at the end of 4 years. We anticipate similar results in a study of an effective chemonucleolytic agent.

CHYMOPAPAIN VERSUS STEROIDS

C. Edmund Graham[24] presented a two-year follow-up of a double-blind study comparing intradiscal injection of chymopapain to hydrocortisone. Satisfactory symptomatic relief was obtained in 45% of 20 chymopapain-treated patients and in only 16% of 19 hydrocortisone-injected patients. In this poorly designed study, 10 of the 20 chymopapain patients had back pain as a primary complaint; seven of the 19 hydrocortisone patients had back pain predominantly. Over half of the hydrocortisone-treated patients were Workmen's Compensation cases, and 12 of the chymopapain-treated patients were on compensation. Poor patient selection could account for the low percentage of satisfactory symptomatic relief in both groups.

The author suggested that chymopapain was superior in efficacy to intradiscal injection of hydrocortisone. This is a very confusing study in that Feffer originally showed that hydrocortisone was more efficacious in patients with back pain as a primary complaint, compared with those with leg pain.[25]

"TRIPLE-BLIND" STUDY

By the summer of 1982, a number of investigators in as many institutions in North America had injected over 120 patients in a triple-blind study comparing the efficacy of Discase to CEI (the original placebo in the first double-blind study) to saline (control). Travenol Laboratories[26] summarized the early results of this study in a new drug application to the FDA. The study was redesigned in accordance with our original recommendations to eliminate unnecessary early code break and to double the dosage of Discase utilized in the original study. In this study, 2 cc (8 mg or 4,000 units) of the enzyme was injected per disc.

Surgery was required for relief of sciatica in 11% of the Discase-injected patients, versus 40% of the CEI patients and 44% of the patients who received saline. Satisfactory results were perceived by 78% of patients in the Discase group, compared with 57% of the CEI group and 22% of the saline group.

Failure to obtain better results with CEI than with saline was not

TABLE 3–4.—URONIC ACID
(μG) RELEASED FROM HUMAN
NUCLEUS PULPOSUS IN VITRO*

Discase	52 ± 8.9
CEI	29 ± 5.6
Saline	27 ± 5.1

*Average of 10 determinations.

surprising, in light of laboratory observations at the University of Miami School of Medicine. We found that Discase released significantly more uronic acid into the supernatant fluid from human nucleus in vitro than did CEI or saline. There were no differences in the amount of uronic acid released by either of the latter two substances (Table 3–4). Uronic acid release is an indirect measurement of the enzymatic breakdown of acid aminoglycan molecules in the nucleus pulposus.

AUSTRALIAN DOUBLE-BLIND STUDY

Between March 1979 and September 1980, several surgeons in Australia performed a double-blind study comparing intradiscal injection of 8 mg of Discase to saline (control) in patients with proved disc displacement causing leg pain. Rob Fraser[27] reported the follow-up results of this study in 1982. Sixty patients between the ages of 16 and 69 who had not responded to 3 weeks of conservative management and who were considered ideal candidates for surgery were studied. Six months after injection, 80% of those treated with Discase had a successful outcome, compared with 57% of those injected with saline. More impressive, twice as many (37%) of the patients injected with saline required surgery for relief in the first 6 months as did those who received Discase (17%). These figures are surprisingly close to those calculated from Weber's study (33% unsatisfactory results in a conservatively treated group, versus 14% unsatisfactory results in a surgically treated group).

PURIFIED CHYMOPAPAIN CONTROLLED STUDY

Travenol Laboratories withdrew the chymopapain IND number from the FDA following the first double-blind study. Subsequently, a group in Illinois started a new company, Smith Laboratories, Inc., to produce and test a "purified" chymopapain for chemonucleolysis. In a double-blind study, they compared Chymodiactin, their preparation of chymopapain, with saline placebo. The study was conducted in seven university medical centers on 108 patients with proved disc displacement at one level, causing leg pain despite at least 2 weeks of bedrest and a total of 6 weeks of conservative treatment. More than 80% of the patients who received the purified chymopapain did not break code and had satisfactory relief of symptoms, compared with 40% in the saline control group.[28]

EPIDURAL STEROIDS

Wiesel, Bernini, and Rothman[29] presented the results of a double-blind study comparing 80 mg of methylprednisolone mixed with lidocaine to saline mixed with lidocaine (control) in the management of 36 patients with proved disc displacement and persistent symptoms of sciatic leg pain despite 3 weeks' bedrest and aspirin prior to entering the study. Twenty-one months following injection, five of the 22 patients (22.7%) who received steroids were "improved," compared with three of the 14 (21.4%) patients who received saline. There was no significant difference in relief of symptoms. The addition of steroids to the epidural injection had no therapeutic value.

The results of this study are pertinent to the chymopapain studies because nearly 22% of the patients still obtained relief despite an epidural injection of saline alone. This is further evidence of the spontaneously expected cure rate from a herniated disc.

It is difficult to compare this and other studies with Weber's study because of variations in the criteria for satisfactory and unsatisfactory results.

COMPARISON OF STUDIES

Patient Selection

In an attempt to compare and correlate the results of various studies to determine the true efficacy of both the enzyme and the utilization technique, one encounters several problems, the first of which is variation in patient selection. Most investigators agree that, in a study design, patients with diagnosed disc herniation resulting in sciatica must have the following symptoms: leg pain greater than back pain, straight leg raising painful at less than 50 degrees, neurologic deficit(s), and a correspondingly positive myelogram consistent with a herniated disc at one level. Most of the uncontrolled studies and a few of the controlled studies did not have these strict criteria for patient selection.

Conservative Care

The problem in conservative care is to determine the point at which further treatment is unlikely to yield results, so that patient suffering

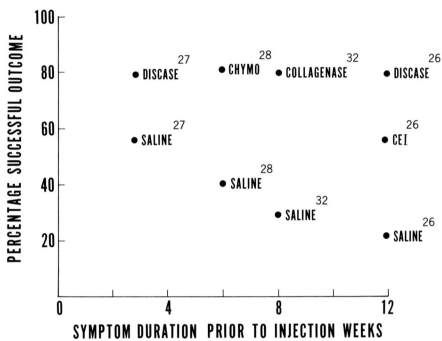

ENZYME COMPARED TO SALINE

Fig 3–1.—Percentage of patients with satisfactory treatment outcome compared with average duration of symptoms (in weeks) before entry into four controlled studies of proved disc displacement. Numbers refer to references at end of chapter.

is not needlessly prolonged. This point is dramatically illustrated by the variations in incidence of satisfactory response to placebo in controlled studies. Despite a high degree of selectivity in these studies, favorable results occurred in 22%–57% of patients receiving a placebo injection (Fig 3–1). We plotted the duration of sciatica before patients were admitted to various studies in relation to the success rate for the various placebos (CEI or saline) and the various injection treatments (chymopapain, collagenase, surgery). The longer the patient had suffered from sciatica (2–12 weeks), the worse the prognosis for the placebos, and the better the prognosis for the active treatments. However, more than 3 months of conservative treatment for disabling pain and neurologic deficit(s) portends a poor prognosis, according to some authorities.[30]

Adequate conservative care includes 2 weeks of bedrest, according to Wiesel and Rothman.[31] Even with strict patient selection criteria which include 2 months of unremitting symptoms and 2 weeks of bedrest, 33% early satisfactory results can be achieved 8 weeks after intradiscal injection of saline.[32]

Long-term follow-up (between 4 and 10 years) in a well-selected series of patients with proved disc displacement shows progressive increase in the incidence of satisfactory results, as well as objective improvement following conservative management.[33]

Outcome of Treatment

Another difficulty in comparing various studies lies in the criteria for determining treatment outcome. Most series follow the criteria established by MacNab in 1971,[34] which are based strictly on the physician's evaluation of the patient's pain, function, and objective findings. MacNab himself[35] grouped his "excellent" and "good" results into a category labeled *successful* and his "fair" and "poor" results into a category labeled *failed* for the purposes of evaluating chemonucleolysis (Table 3–5).

In order to compare the various series and different treatments for symptomatic disc displacement, we considered satisfactory symptomatic relief[36] to include MacNab's "excellent" results (patients did not complain of back or leg pain, had full work and recreational activities, and had improved objective physical findings) and "good" results (patients had some intermittent back and/or leg pain that did not impair their usual activities and had improved objective physical findings). Unsatisfactory results included MacNab's "fair," "poor," and "worse" categories. *Fair* means patients had intermittent or constant pain that affected work and/or recreational activities, and they may or may not have had

TABLE 3–5.—Criteria For Measuring Treatment Outcome

INVESTIGATOR	OUTCOME	CRITERIA
MacNab[35]	Successful	1. Completely free of pain
		2. Minor discomfort, normal activity
	Failed	3. Better but pain interferes with normal activity
		4. No change in symptoms
Brown[36]	Satisfactory symptomatic relief	
	Excellent	1. No pain, full function, objective improvement
	Good	2. Some pain, full function, objective improvement
	Unsatisfactory	
	Fair	3. Some pain, modified activity, ± objective improvement
	Poor	4. Same pain, impaired function, no improvement in signs
	Worse	5. Pain worse, loss of function, increased impairment

improved objective physical findings. *Poor* means no change in pretreatment symptoms, function, or physical findings. *Worse* means patients had increased pain, decreased function, or worsening of objective findings.

Code Break

Results of treatment can be measured by the failure to break code, which is presumed to be a joint decision of the patient and physician based on a favorable outcome of treatment. However, when the treatment is followed by a temporary increase in symptoms (e.g., nerve root inflammation following intradiscal enzyme injection resulting in temporary increase in back and leg pain), code break should not be allowed before a predetermined time. Premature code break absolutely biased the results of the first double-blind study against chymopapain, which caused a greater temporary increase in symptoms than the placebo CEI.[19]

Physical Exam

Improved spinal flexion, straight leg raising, and neurologic deficits are important criteria for determining a physiologic response to treatment. Improvement in these objective parameters, however, does not necessarily mean an improvement in symptoms or function.

Disability

The most sensitive criterion for evaluating treatment outcome, according to a recent study, is the patient's perception of disability as determined by a questionnaire.[37] None of the studies cited here have utilized this technique. I think this is an excellent way of obtaining a holistic measurement of treatment outcome independent of the physician who selects the patients and performs the study. Thus a certain bias is eliminated.

Future Studies

The minimum requirement for measuring efficacy of treatment with a chemonucleolytic agent is a controlled study. Code break rate, objective criteria from physical examinations, and patients' perceptions of pain and disability should be used to measure outcome.

The ease with which the efficacy of collagenase was proved with as few as 30 well-selected patients, utilizing the methods for determining outcome noted above, stands out in marked contrast to the large uncontrolled and controlled trials with chymopapain.

From the numerous well-controlled studies of chymopapain and the

one well-designed study on collagenase, we have concluded that both
enzymes are effective for chemical decompression of displaced discs that
do not respond to adequate conservative care. In my opinion, no further
controlled studies are necessary to prove the efficacy of these enzymes.

CHYMOPAPAIN: PHASE IV

In February 1974, the Canadian Food and Drug Administration au-
thorized the release of chymopapain in Phase IV of its clinical trials,
and the drug also became available in England. John A. McCulloch,
Toronto, became the major consultant for U.S. physicians who referred
patients to Canada for chemonucleolysis. By May 1979, McCulloch had
treated over 2,000 patients, and he published follow-up reports in
1980.[38] He also published the results of his experience with 79 outpa-
tients who had undergone chemonucleolysis.[39] Extrapolating from 1978
figures of 160,000 simple laminectomies done in the United States for
disc excision, McCulloch predicted that outpatient chemonucleolysis
could save up to $500,000,000 per year in medical expenses in the
United States alone.

By August 1982, McCulloch had performed more than 5,000 chymopapain injections under local anesthesia with no permanent morbidity
or mortality.[40] He had successfully managed 15 patients with immediate severe systemic allergic reactions by early administration of epinephrine and intravenous fluids.

Leavitt and his colleagues[41] compared patients treated by chymopapain injection with patients treated by laminectomy, using a multidimensional pain scale. From their measurements over 14 weeks, they
concluded that patients treated with chymopapain do as well as those
treated by laminectomy for back and leg pain. Chymopapain produces
rapid, early improvement, while patients with laminectomy seem to
have a slower rate of healing with respect to pain.

Javid[42] reported his experience with chymopapain in the treatment of
124 patients. At one-year follow-up, 90 (72.6%) of them experienced satisfactory symptomatic relief. After 3 to 6 years, there was no change in
the overall percentage of patients with satisfactory relief of symptoms.
Of patients with no previous back surgery who were not on Workmen's
Compensation, 83.3% showed satisfactory relief in long-term follow-up.
Javid confirmed the work of Wiltse in the one-year follow-up neurologic
examination: 81.6% of patients with prechemonucleolysis weakness had
returned to normal; 65.7% with sensory impairment and 61.8% with
diminished or absent reflexes had returned to normal (see Table 2–3).
Patients who had subsequent laminectomy had no adverse effects from
chymopapain. This had been a consistent finding among all previous
observers.

REFERENCES

1. Crout J.R.: Statement from Bureau of Drugs, U.S. Food and Drug Administration. *J. Neurosurg.* 42:373, 1975.
2. Clark M.A.: Statement from the Office of Scientific Evaluation, U.S. Food
   and Drug Administration. (Position statement on chymopapain.) *J. Neurosurg.* 42:373, 1975.
3. American Association of Neurologic Surgeons: Position Statement on chymopapain. *J. Neurosurg.* 42:373, 1975.
4. World Medical Association: Declaration of Helsinki: Recommendations guiding doctors in clinical research. *J.A.M.A.* 197:31, 1966.
5. Report of the Committee on Chymopapain (Discase). Chicago, American
   Academy of Orthopaedic Surgeons, 1975.
6. Pearce J., Moll J.M., III: Conservative treatment and natural history of
   acute lumbar disc lesions. *J. Neurol. Neurosurg. Psychiatry* 30:13, 1967.
7. Aussman R.K.: Personal communication, 1974.
8. Beecher H.K.: Appraisal of drugs intended to alter subjective responses.
   J.A.M.A. 158:399, 1955.
9. Beecher H.K.: Surgery as placebo: A quantitative study of bias. *J.A.M.A.*
   176:1102, 1957.
10. Cobb L.S. et al.: Evaluation of internal mammary artery ligation by double-
    blind technique. *N. Engl. J. Med.* 260:1115, 1959.
11. Travenol Laboratories: Protocol for double-blind study comparing Discase to
    placebo. 1974.
12. Travenol Laboratories: Statistical analysis and tabulation of data resulting
    from Discase double-blind trial. Intraoffice correspondence, July 28, 1975.
13. Travenol Laboratories: Discase Patient. Attitude and perception study. Re-
    port by Rabin Research Company, June, 1975.
14. Cloud G.A., Doyle J.E., Sanford R.L., et al.: *Final Statistical Analysis of the
    Discase Double-Blind Clinical Trial.* Durfall, Ill., Biostatistical Services
    Dept. Travenol Laboratories, 1976.
15. Reynolds F.C.: Report on double-blind study to the American Academy of
    Orthopaedic Surgeons, Letter, Nov. 7, 1975.
16. Knighton R.S.: Evaluation of the authenticity of the controlled double-blind
    study of chymopapain. Report to Baxter Travenol, 1975.
17. Brown M.D.: Report to Baxter Travenol of the Long-Term (4 years) Tele-
    phone Follow-up of the Double Blind Study. May 12, 1981.
18. Schwetschenau P.R., Ramirez A., Johnston J., et al.: Double-blind evalua-
    tions of intradiscal chymopapain for herniated lumbar discs: Early results.
    J. Neurosurg. 45:622, 1976.
19. Brown M.D., Daroff R.B.: The double-blind study comparing Discase to pla-
    cebo: An editorial comment. *Spine* 2:233, 1977.
20. Martins A.N., Ramirez A., Johnston J., Schwetschenau P.R.: Double-blind
    evaluation of chemonucleolysis for herniated lumbar discs: Late results. *J.
    Neurosurg.* 49:816, 1978.
21. Nordby E.J., Brown M.D.: Present status of chymopapain and chemonucleo-
    lysis. *Clin. Orthop.* 129:79, 1977.
22. Weber H.: An evaluation of conservative and surgical treatment of lumbar
    disc protrusion. *J. Oslo City Hosp.* 20:810, 1970.
23. Weber H.: Lumbar disc herniation: A prospective study of prognostic factors
    including a controlled trial. *J. Oslo City Hosp.* 28:33, 1978.
24. Graham C.E.: Chemonucleolysis: A double-blind study comparing chemo-
    nucleolysis with intradiscal hydrocortisone in the treatment of backache
    and sciatica. *Clin. Orthop.* 117:179, 1976.

25. Feffer H.L.: Treatment of low back and sciatic pain by the injection of hydrocortisone into degenerated intervertebral discs. *J. Bone Joint Surg.* 38-A:585, 1956.

26. Travenol Laboratories: *The Clinical Summary of New Drug Application to the FDA—Safety and Efficacy.* Deerfield, Ill., Baxter Travenol Laboratories, 1982.

27. Fraser R.D.: Chymopapain for the treatment of intervertebral disc prolapse: A double-blind study. Paper presented to the International Society for the Study of the Lumbar Spine, Toronto, June 1982.

28. Nordby E.: Personal communication, August 1982.

29. Wiesel S., Bernini P., Rothman R.: Effectiveness of epidural steroids in the treatment of sciatica—A double-blind clinical trial. Paper presented to the International Society for the Study of the Lumbar Spine, Toronto, June 1982.

30. Hakelius A.: Prognosis in sciatica. *Acta Orthop. Scand.* (suppl.) 129:1, 1970.

31. Wiesel S.W., Rothman R.H.: Acute low back pain: An objective analysis of conservative therapy. *Clin. Orthop.* 143:290, 1979.

32. Bromley J.: Clinical and double-blind studies concerning collagenase. Paper presented to Deidesheimes Gespräch, Deidesheim, Germany, 1982.

33. Weber H.: Lumbar disc herniation—A controlled prospective study with ten years' observation. Paper presented to the International Society for the Study of the Lumbar Spine, Toronto, 1982.

34. MacNab I.: Negative disc exploration. *J. Bone Joint Surg.* 53-A:891, 1971.

35. MacNab I.: Chemonucleolysis. *Clin. Neurosurg.* 20:183, 1973.

36. Brown M.D.: Chemonucleolysis with Discase: Technique, results, case reports. *Spine* 1:115, 1976.

37. Roland M., Morris R.: A study of the natural history of back pain. I: Development of a reliable and sensitive measure of disability in low back pain. *Spine,* accepted for publication 1983.

38. McCulloch J.A.: Chemonucleolysis: Experience with 2,000 cases. *Clin. Orthop.* 146:128, 1980.

39. McCulloch J., Ferguson J.: Outpatient chemonucleolysis. *Spine* 6:606, 1981.

40. McCulloch J.: Personal communication, August 1982.

41. Leavitt F., Garron D., Whisler W., et al.: A comparison of patients treated by chymopapain and laminectomy for low back pain using a multidimensional pain scale. *Clin. Orthop.* 146:136, 1980.

42. Javid M.: Treatment of herniated lumbar disc syndrome with chymopapain. *J.A.M.A.* 243:2043, 1980.

4 / Collagenase

In 1953, Ines Mandl and coworkers[1] reported the isolation of collagenase from *Clostridium histolyticum*. They had biochemical and electron microscopic proof of this enzyme's specificity to catalyze native undenatured collagen. By 1958, Mandl and coworkers[2] had purified the collagenase by continuous curtain electrophoresis. One of the earliest clinical uses of this highly purified bacterial collagenase was in ointments for debridement of burns.

APPLICATION TO DISCOLYSIS

Bernard J. Sussman[3] was the first to recommend the application of collagenase for intervertebral "discolysis." He suggested this enzyme as an alternative to chymopapain because of his fears about the enzyme's toxicity and the adverse reactions encountered in the Phase I studies. The rationale for the use of collagenase to dissolve discs was based on the high collagen content of degenerated herniated nucleus pulposus and annulus fibrosus.

Sussman demonstrated the enzymatic digestion of human nucleus pulposus and fibrocartilage removed at surgery and the lack of dissolution of small arteries, bone, and articular cartilage removed at autopsy. He stated that the selective action of collagenase against fibrocartilage in nucleus pulposus, with sparing of hyaline cartilage and mature fibrosus tissue such as the anterior longitudinal ligament, made it an ideal substance for "discolysis."

In 1969, Sussman used collagenase in vivo to dissolve nucleus pulposus in dogs; he found no adverse systemic reactions to the enzyme.[4] He suggested later (1971) that collagenase was a better agent for discolysis because it had a higher dissolution effect on nucleus pulposus than chymopapain.[5]

Collagenase specifically degrades collagen and does not affect noncollagenous protein or cell membranes. It is rapidly inactivated by serum and is bound to the substrate, according to Sussman. Clinical experience with collagenase in burn ointments, in facilitating transplantation of allograft teeth, and as a cell dispersion agent in tissue cultures suggested the gentle nature of this enzyme with respect to cellular toxicity. Comparing collagenase to chymopapain, Sussman stated that the former was a safer agent. Moreover, he thought that any injected collagenase leaking from the disc and coming into contact with the dura would not injure it because the dura is protected by a cellular layer which is not affected by collagenase. Inadvertent intrathecal injection of collagenase was thought to be potentially less harmful than chymopapain to the neural elements, due to the protective mesenchymal cellular barrier of the pia-arachnoid. He also thought that the capillary microvasculature was protected because of the endothelial cell lining.

CRITICISM OF COLLAGENASE

In response to Sussman's criticism of chymopapain, Paul Garvin published a paper in 1974 on the toxicity of collagenase.[6] He used crude collagenase from Worthington Laboratories, stating that, based on activity, there was no significant difference in the acute intravenous toxicity of the crude and purified forms. In rabbits, Garvin found that 100 units or less per disc caused dissolution of the nucleus pulposus, with no effect on the annulus fibrosus. He found that intrathecal doses of 19 units per kilogram in dogs caused death. (The weights of the dogs were not given.) He noted intrathecal toxicity in the form of hemorrhage, reminiscent of that seen with chymopapain. It is difficult to understand the significance of this and other studies on both enzymes concerning intrathecal toxic dose versus effective disc dissolution dose because of variations in the sources of the enzyme studied, the different animals used, and the inconsistent calculation of dosage in units or in milligrams per kilogram.

PHARMACOLOGY OF COLLAGENASE

John W. Bromley, an orthopedic surgeon, and Harold Stern, a researcher, were instrumental in the commercial development of highly purified *C. histolyticum* collagenase in a small company called Advance Biofactures. In 1970, Stern learned about the possible application of collagenase to discolysis at an intradisciplinary symposium.[7] Stern and Bromley tested the efficacy of purified collagenase for intervertebral disc dissolution.

In 1980, Bromley, along with other collaborators, presented the results of studies on the enzyme's dissolution effect in dogs, monkeys, and humans.[8] They found the minimum effective discolysis dose of collagenase to be 315 units per disc in the dog and monkey. Extrapolating from studies on human disc material removed at surgery, they determined the effective dose per disc for humans to be 300–600 units.

Toxicity studies showed a relative margin of safety with respect to intradiscal, intravenous, intraperitoneal, paraspinal, and extradural injections of collagenase in the dog and monkey, compared with the effective dissolution dose within the disc. However, the margin of safety for intrathecal injection in dogs and monkeys was relatively low. The effective intradiscal dissolution dose for dogs was 315 units per disc, they exhibited neurologic change from 800 units injected intrathecally. Two thousand units injected intrathecally induced paraplegia in every instance. Between two and six times the effective intradiscal dose is toxic when injected intrathecally in dogs and monkeys. Between one and three times the effective intradiscal dose of chymopapain is toxic when injected intrathecally in monkeys. Chymopapain appears to have a more immediate effect on rupture of the microvasculature, but collagenase seems to have a similar effect.

According to Bromley, sensitization tests in guinea pigs showed that Nucleolysin (Advance Biofacture's collagenase) was not antigenic. A word of caution in this regard: similar studies on chymopapain showed it not to be antigenic either![9]

PHASE I TRIALS

In 1981, a clinical follow-up on the first 29 patients treated by intradiscal injection of collagenase was reported by Bernard Sussman, Howard University Hospital; Washington, D.C., John Bromley, St. Joseph's Hospital Medical Center, Paterson, N.J.; and Jaime Gomez, Neurologic Institute of Colombia, Bogotá.[10]

The initial report was based on 29 adult patients between the ages of 21 and 60 with back and leg pain unresponsive to conservative therapy for more than 60 days. Patients with limited straight leg raising, neurologic deficit, positive myelogram with a single disc herniation, and without a history of previous surgery, severe neurologic deficit, pregnancy, arthritis, previous exposure to topical collagenase, or severe psychosomatic problems were selected for the initial clinical trial. Complete relief or "noticeable amelioration of pain" occurred in 63% of patients, and an additional 21% reported moderate relief of pain. Four patients (14%) failed to respond, underwent surgery, and were found to have an extruded disc fragment in the spinal canal as the reason for failure. The clinical course in these patients differs from that reported for patients injected with chymopapain. That is, the majority of patients do not experience relief of leg pain within the first few hours after injection. Some patients had increased back pain and muscle spasms, which lasted from 3 days to 2 weeks. Most patients showed narrowing of the discs injected; and, in one patient who had recurrent symptoms 2 months after injection, a repeat myelogram showed resolution of the myelographic defect.

Between March 1979 and June 1980, 82 patients were injected intradiscally with collagenase. Thirty-six of these patients were treated at the Neurologic Institute in Bogotá by Gomez. The remaining 46 were treated at St. Joseph's Hospital, Paterson, N. J. by Bromley, who presented the study results in the spring of 1982.[11] He noted a clinical course characterized by a gradual loss of leg pain over several weeks after injection. Approximately 25% of the patients had markedly increased back pain and muscle spasms, which lasted from 1 to 10 days. Patients had a gradual improvement in neurologic deficits that paralleled their clinical improvement. Patients who did not improve within 6 weeks after injection were considered failures, and most went on to surgery. Of the 82 patients treated, four received 300 units of Neucleolysin per disc; only 1 of these four had good results. The remaining 78 patients received between 500 and 600 units of Neucleolysin per disc. All patients were injected at one level, one patient at L3-4, 54 at L4-5, and 27 at the L5-S1 disc space.

Results in 76 of the patients (80.4%) were classified as excellent or good, four patients (4.9%) improved and were classified as fair, and 22 (14.7%) had poor results. Ten of the 12 patients who underwent surgery were found to have undissolved extruded disc material as a cause for failure. All patients showed at least 40% to 60% narrowing of the interspace 4–6 weeks after injection despite 300 or 600 units of injected enzyme, even though the dose varied widely.

The only complication was a transient increase in dorsiflexion weakness in two patients. It resolved spontaneously after approximately 4 weeks, with full recovery of motor strength and a good end result. No systemic or local toxicity and no neurologic reactions were noted. Bromley stated that disc extrusion and/or sequestration occurs in about 13% of patients in surgical disc series. Therefore, the 84.6% success rate indicates the high efficacy of collagenase to dissolve herniated discs and relieve symptoms when it can reach the offending tissue.

PHASE II TRIALS

On the basis of data from initial clinical trials with collagenase, an application was submitted to the FDA for a double-blind study; it was approved June 23, 1980. Between June 1980 and November 1981, 30 patients were studied; analysis of the results showed significant difference in outcome when collagenase was compared with placebo.

Only patients between 20 and 60 years of age who had had unremitting back and leg pain for at least 60 days that had not responded to conservative therapy (including 2 weeks of bedrest) were accepted into the study. Other criteria were: leg pain as the predominant complaint associated with limited straight leg raising, a single-level disc herniation confirmed by myelography, no previous surgery, no serious neurologic deficit (e.g., complete foot drop). Patients who had previously been exposed to collagenase ointment, were pregnant, had open epiphyses, or had other contraindications for injection were excluded. Patients had to have as their sole diagnosis a disc herniation syndrome. For example, patients with systemic disorders such as diabetes or psychogenic disease were excluded. The technique for injection was identical to that of previous series with chymopapain, except that the injection was not preceded by a discogram. Patients were encouraged not to break code merely to satisfy curiosity.

The evaluation of treatment was based upon code break rate, patients' estimate of pain, and investigators' evaluations. After 30 patients were treated with this protocol and 8 weeks of follow-up had intervened, there was such a dramatic difference in code break (66% of 15 patients treated with placebo broke code and 14% of the collagenase-treated patients broke code [$P < 0.01$]) that no further patients were enlisted in the protocol. Eight weeks after injection, 80% of the collagenase-treated patients had a successful result, as opposed to 30% of the placebo-treated patients, which was statistically significant ($P < 0.005$). There was a highly significant difference in the patients' estimate of pain when comparing placebo with Nucleolysin. The investigators' evaluation of 8 weeks found that forward flexion and straight leg raising were significantly better following collagenase treatment.[12]

In December 1981, the results of this study were reviewed by the FDA, and Advance Biofactures was given permission to use Nucleolysin in a Phase III open clinical trial.

AUTHOR'S EXPERIENCE WITH COLLAGENASE

The Human Research Committee at the University of Miami School of Medicine approved the protocol for a Phase II double-blind study of collagenase in the spring of 1981. The study was completed prior to selection of any patients for the controlled study. We were subsequently approved for Phase III trials and have treated 23 patients to date. Thus far, 13 have had excellent or good results, and 6 patients have had fair or poor results; three of the latter patients have submitted to surgery. One patient had an extruded disc, one patient a sequestrated disc, and a third patient had a bulging annulus fibrosus as the reasons for failure. There has been no evidence of a deleterious effect on surrounding epidural venous plexus, longitudinal ligaments, dura, or nerve root sleeve coverings. Four patients are within 6 weeks of injection; 10 of the 23 patients have had severe postinjection pain lasting for 7 to 21 days, which is the most common adverse reaction experienced thus far.

CURRENT EXPERIENCE

To date, approximately 200 patients have been treated with collagenase with no systemic sensitivity reaction. We think that the drug has a good margin of safety, comparing the effective intradiscal dissolution dose with the toxic intrathecal dose, and a comparable or reduced risk of sensitivity reaction. For this reason, we think that it is an appropriate alternative drug for chemonucleolysis. Postinjection pain, both local and referred, is more severe with collagenase than with chymopapain, in my experience.

A further comparison of collagenase with chymopapain is made in Chapter 8.

REFERENCES

1. Mandl I., MacLennan J., Howes E.: Isolation and characterization of proteinase and collagenase from *C. histolyticum*. *J. Clin. Invest.* 32:1312, 1953.
2. Mandl I., Zipper H., Ferguson L.T.: *Clostridium histolyticum* collagenase: Its purification and properties. *Arch. Biochem. Biophys.* 4:465, 1958.
3. Sussman B.J.: Intervertebral discolysis with collagenase. *J. Natl. Med. Assoc.* 60:184, 1968.
4. Sussman B.J., Mann M.: Experimental intervertebral discolysis with collagenase. *J. Neurosurg.* 31:628, 1969.
5. Sussman B.J.: Experimental intervertebral discolysis. A critique of collagenase and chymopapain applications. *Clin. Orthop.* 80:181, 1971.
6. Garvin P.J.: Toxicity of collagenase: The relation to enzyme therapy of disc herniation. *Clin. Orthop.* 101:286, 1974.
7. Mandl I.: Collagenase. Lecture at Interdisciplinary Symposium on Collagenase, Columbia University College of Physicians and Surgeons. *Science* 169:1234, 1970.
8. Bromley J., Hirst J., Osman M., et al.: Collagenase: An experimental study of intervertebral disc dissolution. *Spine* 5:126, 1980.
9. Smith L., Brown J.E.: Treatment of lumbar intervertebral disc lesions by direct injection of chymopapain. *J. Bone Joint Surg.* 49-B:502, 1967.
10. Sussman B., Bromley J., Gomez J.: Injection of collagenase in the treatment of herniated lumbar disk. *J.A.M.A.* 245:730, 1981.
11. Bromley J.: Intervertebral discolysis with collagenase. Paper presented to Deidesheimes Gespräch, Deidesheim, Germany, May 8, 1982.
12. Bromley J., Santaro A., Cohen P., et al.: Double-blind evaluation of collagenase injected for herniated lumbar discs. Paper presented to Deidesheimes Gespräch, Deidesheim, Germany, May 8, 1982.

5 / Indications for Chemonucleolysis

JOHN O'CONNELL stated, "The greatest problem is not diagnosis but deciding upon the correct treatment in each case. The natural history of lumbago and sciatica has not been altered by the discovery of the common cause, and the tendency to spontaneous recovery remains as strong as it has been down the centuries."[1] The wisdom of this statement is illustrated by the work of Hitselberger and Witten,[2] who demonstrated that the mere existence of a herniated lumbar disc does not necessarily mean the patient is suffering pain or disability. They found myelographic defects consistent with disc displacement in the lumbar spine in 37% of 300 patients studied for acoustic neuromas. The patients had no history of back injuries, back pain, or radiculopathy. Their myelographic abnormalities were graded from mild (a deformity of a nerve root sleeve) to severe (a complete block). One asymptomatic patient had a complete block, and 19 patients (6%) had a nearly complete block. Fifty of the patients (17%) had a defect consistent with a significant lateral disc herniation.

Of any consecutive group of patients with leg pain caused by disc displacement, 70% will spontaneously improve with time and conservative care, and will require no further treatment.[3] Two months' elapsed time from the onset of the attack and at least 2 weeks of bedrest constitute adequate conservative care. During this time, the patient should show continual improvement, which means that pain becomes either mild or absent or, if present, intermittent and undisabling. The patient should be able to return to work by the end of 2 months, and, if the pain recurs, should lose less than 4 weeks' work per year as a result of these attacks. There should be progressively fewer physical findings.

Candidates for chemonucleolysis should be selected from the 30% of patients that do not improve with time and rest. Of this group, some will have already suffered for more than 2 months without relief and will have already self-imposed bedrest or limited activity for more than 2 weeks before seeking medical care. For these patients, no further conservative care is indicated, and chemonucleolysis or surgery should be offered if no contraindications exist. A small percentage of this group will present with objective neurologic findings indicative of physical impairment that requires immediate surgical decompression.

IDEAL CANDIDATE

Chemical excision by intradiscal injection of an enzyme is indicated in the patient who is an ideal candidate for *elective* surgical disc excision. The technique should not be used when a delay of 4–6 weeks in obtaining results might be deleterious to the health of the patient (e.g., in cauda equina syndrome). Surgical decompression offers immediate relief of nerve compression, whereas chemonucleolysis with either enzyme may take some time for results to occur.[4]

IDEAL PHYSICIAN

Intradiscal enzyme injection should be done only by qualified orthopedists and neurosurgeons who have a special interest in spinal disorders. They should have some advanced instruction in the indications and hands-on technique involved in chemonucleolysis and be fully trained to manage patients who do not obtain relief.

INFORMED CONSENT

It is difficult to moderate one's enthusiasm for a treatment, particularly when the rationalization is that it affords the patient less risk than surgery and the ability to avoid an incision. However, the patient should be as fully informed as the physician and must participate in the selection of treatment before chemonucleolysis is indicated.

Chemonucleolysis is indicated only when the patient has been fully informed of the nature, benefit, risks, and alternatives of care (including an explanation of the natural history of the disease). Approximately 50% of the time, the symptoms will ameliorate spontaneously if the patient can wait. The patient should also be informed that, in the majority of instances, the pain is not harmful and will not lead to increased damage. It is surprising how many patients will choose to continue a conservative treatment regimen when told these facts.

SMITH'S INDICATIONS

Lyman Smith found that 82 of 100 patients improved markedly following chemonucleolysis with chymopapain between 1967 and 1968. Prior to injection, the patients had leg pain that failed to respond to adequate conservative treatment. He wrote, "I am a little embarrassed to admit that the percentage of marked improvement in my last 100 cases graded at least nine months postinjection has risen to 93%. Why the considerable betterment in statistics in the intervening 5 years? In that period there has been no change in the technique of procedure, the dosage of enzyme, or the methodology of postinjection care. The prime change has been in my own hard-heartedness and selfish decision as to the patients' motivation or lack of it."[5]

The best risks for chemonucleolysis are those patients who have not responded to adequate conservative care for proven symptomatic disc displacement and who are candidates for laminectomy and disc excision.

If one restricts the use of chymopapain to the patient who has had unremitting symptoms for more than 60 days, has not responded to at least 2 weeks of bedrest, has leg pain predominating, has significantly limited straight leg raising, neurologic deficit(s), and a correspondingly positive myelogram and/or CAT scan, a high percentage of excellent and good results can be obtained.

CASE 1 (Fig 5–1).—A 40-year-old male, a manufacturer, had a 5-year history of lumbago and insidious onset of left leg pain 2 months prior to examination on May 20, 1975. He had been in bed at home for 3 weeks, and the leg pain was getting worse. In addition to positive straight leg

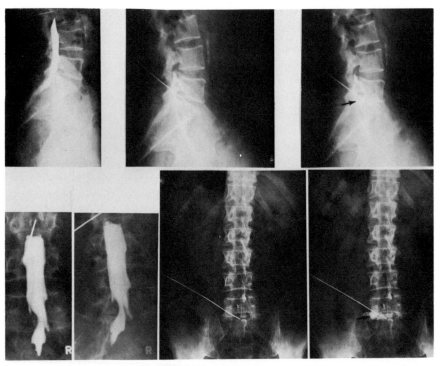

Fig 5–1.—Anterior and posterior roentgenograms of a Pantopaque myelogram *(left)*, needle placement in lumbosacral disc space *(middle)*, and discogram *(right)*, demonstrating a large, lateral extradural defect consistent with herniated fifth lumbar disc, which has been visualized on the discogram with 60% iothalamate.

raising of 20 degrees on the left side with pain into the calf, there was no left Achilles tendon reflex and no posterior tibial reflex. There were two plus reflexes on the right. Plain x-rays showed a calcified abdominal aorta. Peripheral pulses were normal. On May 22, the patient underwent a Pantopaque myelogram, which showed a large extradural defect at L-5 on the left, consistent with a herniated nucleus pulposus. Cerebral spinal fluid protein level was 58 mg%. On May 23, a discogram was performed at L5-S1, which showed filling of the herniated disc corresponding to the extradural defect at the level noted on the myelogram. Upon injection of 2 ml of 60% iothalamate, the patient had a reproduction of his back and left leg pain. After 15 minutes, 1 cc of fluid containing 4 mg of chymopapain was injected intradiscally. Ten minutes after the injection, the patient had relief of left leg pain. He was observed for 5 days in the hospital and walked easily without leg pain but with some increase in back pain. He did not require medication. The patient returned to work 3 weeks after injection. At follow-up 6 weeks after injection, straight leg raising on the left at 60 degrees showed tight hamstrings but no pain. The left Achilles tendon reflex and the left posterior tibial reflex had returned; both were equal to the right-side reflexes. A 4-year follow-up showed the patient had an excellent result, with complete relief of left leg pain and back pain.

AGE LIMITATION

During investigational clinical trials, chemonucleolysis was limited to patients between the ages of 21 and 65.

There are no contraindications to the use of chymopapain in patients younger than 18 or older than 65. Young patients have more proteoglycans in the nucleus pulposus than older persons[6] and therefore should theoretically be better candidates for chymopapain. Nordby injected a 13-year-old patient with excellent results.[7] Wiltse's group demonstrated that 12% of treatment failures occurred in patients in the second and third decade of life, compared with 29% in the fourth and fifth decades.[8] One would expect chymopapain to be more efficacious than collagenase in younger patients. Conversely, patients over 65 have more collagen in their discs;[9] therefore, collagenase should theoretically give better results in the older age group.

In studies where rabbits received intravascular injections of crude papain, depletion of the proteoglycans from the open epiphysis was noted in immature animals. This observation is only theoretically significant when it comes to treating young patients with chymopapain because active enzyme has not been found in the bloodstream following intradiscal injection. Either chymopapain is immediately bound to the matrix substrate of the disc, or the portion that escapes into the bloodstream is inactivated by serum α_2 macroglobulins of the plasma.[10]

I would not place any age restriction on the use of chymopapain for chemonucleolysis. Age-related data on collagenase are not yet available.

DISC DISPLACEMENT CAUSING BACK PAIN VERSUS LEG PAIN

Wiltse's group reviewed 323 patients with various combinations of back and leg pain.[8] Of patients whose back pain was more intense than leg pain, 84.3% obtained satisfactory relief, but Wiltse is careful to point out that this was a carefully selected group of patients who had undergone prolonged conservative care, had normal psychological profiles, and had a central disc displacement proved by myelogram. A primary complaint of back pain secondary to central disc displacement does not contraindicate chemonucleolysis. It is imperative, however, when treating these patients to be certain of the differential diagnosis. A negative bone scan, normal sedimentation rate, and a spinal fluid protein level under 70 mg%,[11] as well as a confirming metrizamide myelogram and CAT scan, are all prerequisites to injecting a patient whose primary complaint is back pain in order to confirm the diagnosis of central disc displacement and rule out the numerous other causes of lumbago (Table 5–1).

TABLE 5–1.—Differential Diagnosis of Low Back Pain
and/or Sciatica From Disc Displacement

Degenerative disc disease	{ Mechanical insufficiency
Spondylolysis	{ Low back pain
Spondylolisthesis	
Spinal stenosis	
Facet joint osteoarthritis	
Metabolic bone disease	
Paget's disease	
Osteopenia, pathologic fracture	
Tumors	
Metastatic from	
Breast	
Prostate	
Primary bone	
Multiple myeloma	
Neurogenic	
Ependymoma	
Neurofibroma	
Infections	
Pyogenic vertebral osteomyelitis	
Disc space infection	
Tuberculosis	
Herpes zoster (shingles)	
Traumatic acute low back sprain	
Psychogenic regional pain disturbance	
Vascular (aortic) aneurysm	
Urogenic (pyelonephritis)	
Viscerogenic (regional enteritis)	
Diabetic neuropathy	

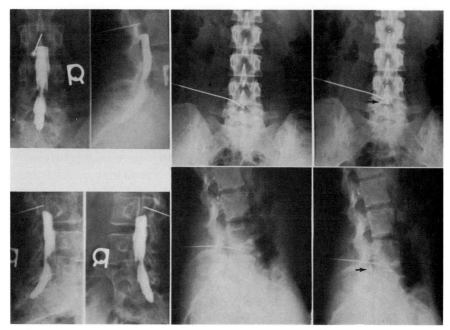

Fig 5–2.—Roentgenograms of various views of Pantopaque myelograms: extradural defect, fourth lumbar interspace; note central herniated nucleus pulposus. Anterior, posterior, and lateral roentgenograms of needle placement and discogram show a central herniated nucleus pulposus at the L4–5 interspace.

CASE 2 (Fig 5–2).—A 25-year old female developed severe low back and bilateral leg pain, the left side being worse than the right, 7 weeks prior to admission to the University of Miami Hospital and Clinics. The back pain began after a karate lesson. Three weeks before admission, the patient developed severe left leg pain and had some relief of the back pain. Physical examination revealed a sciatic list to the left of 20 degrees, a positive straight leg raising on the left at 30 degrees, and contralateral positive straight leg raising at 60 degrees on the right that produced pain in the left leg. In addition to a depressed left Achilles tendon reflex, there was moderate weakness of the extensor hallucis longus and peroneal muscles on the left. There was decreased sensation from pinprick in the first sacral nerve root distribution of the left foot. A Pantopaque myelogram demonstrated a large central disc between the fourth and fifth lumbar interspace. Spinal fluid protein level was 40 mg%. At discography, 1.5 cc of Conray was injected and the patient complained of a reproduction of her pain. A lateral x-ray demonstrated flow of contrast dye into the spinal canal in a configuration consistent with the extradural defect noted on the myelogram. One milliliter of fluid containing 4 mg of chymopapain (Discase) was injected into the fourth lumbar disc on March 28, 1975. Within 30 seconds, the patient complained of tingling around her mouth, perineal and perianal region which lasted for 3 minutes. The reaction was transient and not associated with a change in blood pressure or other systemic or cutaneous manifestations. The patient was discharged from the hospital on March 30, walking comfortably. She had not required any narcotic medication during the observation period. The patient returned to work as a lab technician 2 weeks following the injection and to full recreational activities 3 months after injection. Six years later, she remains fully active at work and recreational activities, experiencing only occasional low backache. She has not required any further treatment. We agree with her perception that she had an excellent result.

RADICULOPATHY DIAGNOSIS

Pain Drawing

People usually have difficulty describing their pain, but patients can express their complaints very well by using a pain drawing.[12] With such a drawing, it is easy to localize various descriptions of pain and other abnormal sensations using symbols on an anterior and posterior silhouette of the body. For example, patients suffering from acute radiculopathy secondary to a herniated disc will depict their pain by placing pain symbols in an anatomically accurate radicular distribution (Fig 5–3,A).

Idiopathic low back pain syndromes secondary to facet osteoarthritis, segmental instability, or discogenic pain will be characterized by symbols for aching sensations in a sclerotogenous pain referred pattern (Fig 5–4). The pain drawing is not as specific for this group of patients as it is for those suffering from radiculopathy.

Psychogenic regional pain disturbances are easily diagnosed by observing the drawing of a patient who suffers from one of these behavioral disorders. One picture literally says a thousand words for these patients (Fig 5–5).

The serial pain drawing is also an excellent method of documenting the response to treatment (see Fig 5–3,B).

History of Herniated Disc

A history of intermittent chronic backache followed by a twisting maneuver and popping sensation in the low back with subsequent pain referral into the leg is characteristic of acute lumbar disc displacement.[13] When the patient states that the onset of leg pain coincides with relief from back pain and this history accompanies an anatomical pain drawing consistent with radiculopathy, you can be certain of the diagnosis of a herniated disc.

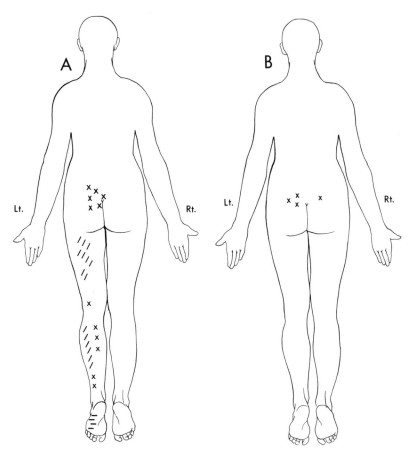

Fig 5–3.—Posterior silhouettes with symbols depicting various sensations such as stabbing //, numbness =, pins and needles O, and aching XX, placed by the patient before *(A)* and 8 weeks after *(B)* chemonucleolysis for first sacral radiculopathy secondary to fifth lumbar disc displacement.

Ninety-five percent of the time, patients with lumbar radiculopathy secondary to disc displacement complain of pain, and only rarely do they present with weakness without pain. The patient with paresis in the absence of pain should alert the physician to a possible tumor.[14]

Sleep Disturbance

The radicular pain of disc herniation is described as a "toothache-like" pain, aggravated by activity and relieved by rest. However, sleep disturbance is a fairly common symptom caused by radicular pain. Patients may have some difficulty getting to sleep and may be awakened with leg pain, which is relieved by walking. In cases of disc displacement, the

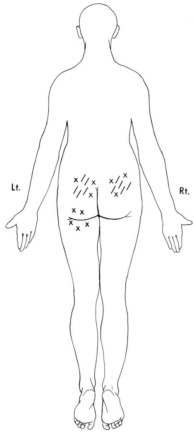

Lt.   Rt.

Fig 5–4.—Posterior silhouette with symbols placed by the patient depicting various sensations typical of sclerotogenous pain referral from acute facet joint osteoarthritis.

sleep disturbance tends to improve with a few days of bedrest. Progressive sleep disturbance despite adequate bedrest should lead one to suspect a space-taking lesion (tumor or infection).[15]

Mechanical Pain

Segmental insufficiency resulting in mechanical low back pain secondary to degenerative disc disease is a diagnosis of exclusion.[16] Patients usually state that they have predominant back pain rather than leg pain. Pain can be referred to the groin, buttocks, and lateral thighs; it is aggravated by activity and relieved by rest. Standing, sitting, or leaning forward for any period of time aggravates the pain. Patients have difficulty pushing or pulling objects, straightening up from a bent

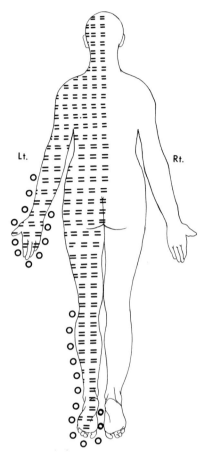

Fig 5–5.—Posterior silhouette with symbols placed by the patient depicting various sensations in a distribution typical of psychogenic regional pain disturbance.

position, and twisting. Lifting is impaired by pain, as well as sitting in a stressful position—for example, on the floor. Recurrent acute attacks of low back pain, brought on by any activity and relieved by rest, and low back fatigue toward the end of the day are also symptoms of mechanical insufficiency.

Plain x-rays may show degenerative spondylolisthesis or a pars interarticularis defect, with or without spondylolisthesis. The diagnosis may also be confirmed by standing stress films, which show displacement of one vertebra over another or angulation greater than 15 degrees.[17]

Chronic low-grade back pain of a mechanical nature is a relative contraindication to chemonucleolysis, even if it is associated with a painful disc displacement. Patients who suffer from this combination of symptoms from degenerative intervertebral joints require surgical decompression and arthrodesis. We do not think that chemonucleolysis with either enzyme enhances stability of the motion segment unit (intervertebral joint complex).

Systemic Illness

The medical history is significant in selecting an ideal candidate for chemonucleolysis. One should avoid patients with a history of previous thromboembolic disease, diabetes mellitus, alcoholism, and other debil-

TABLE 5–2.—CONTRAINDICATIONS FOR CHEMONUCLEOLYSIS

With Chymopapain
  History of allergy to papaya, meat tenderizer, or chymopapain
  Prior injection with chymopapain
With Collagenase
  Exposure to burn ointment containing collagenase
  Previous serious wound infection
  Previous collagenase injection
Severe Neurologic Deficit
  Cauda equina syndrome
  Flail foot
  Gastrocnemius-soleus paralysis (poor pushoff)
  Gluteus paralysis (positive Trendelenburg's sign)
  Quadriceps paralysis
  Neurogenic bladder
  Neurogenic bowel
  Bilateral lower extremity paresis
  Progressive neurologic deficit
Coincidental Diagnosis
  Pregnancy
  Ankylosing spondylitis
  Rheumatoid arthritis
  Poor general health (alcohol, medication, or drug abuse)
  Insulin-dependent diabetes mellitus
Differential Diagnosis
  Suspicion of spinal cord tumor
  Spinal fluid protein level higher than 80 mg%
  Suspected disc space infection and/or
  Vertebral osteomyelitis
  Metastatic cancer
X-ray Findings
  Complete or almost complete block myelogram
  Cervical discs
  Thoracic discs
  Spondylolisthesis (relative contraindication)
  Disc space inaccessible by lateral route
  Spinal stenosis
  Mechanical insufficiency (gas shadow disc space, translation on stress films)
  Intrathecal and/or intravascular flow of contrast at discography
Psychogenic Regional Pain Disturbance Associated With
  Severe depression
  Hysterical symptoms and signs
  Psychosis
  Severe neurosis (hypochondriasis)

itating disease such as chronic hepatitis, rheumatoid arthritis, or malignancy. Patients with a history of multiple previous operations, accidents, illnesses, or multiple allergies have a poor prognosis in chemonucleolysis or any other invasive procedure. Patients with disorders that mimic symptoms of painful lumbar disc displacement should be ruled out as candidates for chemonucleolysis (Table 5–2).

Infection

A recent history of urinary tract infection or diagnostic procedures involving the urinary tract may be an important clue to a hematogenous disc space infection. Pain that results from disc space infection is usually localized to the area of the disc involved and is progressive and unremitting. Early in the diagnosis, blood studies (WBC, sedimentation rate) and x-rays (plain film and bone scan) may be negative. However, if adequate time for conservative care has elapsed (2 months), the tests usually become positive. Suspected disc space infection and/or vertebral osteomyelitis is an absolute contraindication for enzyme injection.

Allergy History

The medical history should include a listing of multiple previous allergies or specific allergy to papain, meat tenderizer, or prior exposure to chymopapain, all of which are contraindications to the use of this enzyme. A history of cutaneous allergic reaction to burn ointments containing collagenase contraindicates the use of the enzyme. Patients previously injected with collagenase should also not be re-exposed by a repeat injection of that enzyme.

SOCIOGENIC AND PSYCHOGENIC CONSIDERATIONS

Hysteria and Hypochondriasis

Certain psychogenic syndromes coinciding with proved painful lumbar disc displacement constitute a miserable prognosis for relief, according to Wiltse and Rocchio.[18] When the patient exhibits strong hysterical and hypochondriacal symptoms confirmed by average combined scores of more than 70 on the Minnesota Multiphasic Personality Inventory Hys and Hyc scales, the prognosis for a successful outcome is poor.

Nonorganic Physical Findings

We have found that patients with any of the nonorganic physical findings described by Waddell and his associates[19] are very difficult to diagnose accurately with respect to significant organic findings, let alone treat by an invasive method. Surprisingly, we have never encountered a patient with more than two nonorganic physical findings who also had hard organic findings. We theorize that the patient with severe organic pain is suffering enough already to satisfy anxiety, hysteria, and/or hypochondriacal tendencies. The nonorganic physical findings encountered most often are: giving way while toe walking (patients with real pain cannot do this; it requires good coordination and muscle control), loss of sensation over an entire extremity in an nonanatomical distribution, active resistance to straight leg raising, and superficial spinal pain and tenderness to palpation.

The typical patient that we see with a combination of these findings has frequently been out of work because of job-related injuries for more than 6 months, is using narcotic medications, depends on disability income for a livelihood, has seen numerous practitioners who have noted few positive physical findings, has undergone a maximum number of treatment modalities.

These easily recognized patients (typical pain drawing, difficult history of present illness, typical medical history, nonorganic physical findings, and negative confirmatory tests) are not good candidates for further treatment of any nature, let alone chemonucleolysis. They require detoxification, increased activity, rapid settlement of claims, and encouragement not to seek further medical care other than periodic follow-up examinations to rule out coincidental or new disease and to maintain a rehabilitative course toward re-entry into the mainstream of life.

SPINAL STENOSIS

Neurogenic or vascular claudication usually implies a diagnosis other than disc herniation. Unilateral or bilateral leg pain brought on by activity and relieved by rest is most commonly caused by central and/or foramenal spinal stenosis.[20]

It is helpful to differentiate radiculopathy secondary to disc displacement from neurogenic claudication secondary to spinal stenosis on a patholphysiologic basis. The former results from a mechanical distortion of the nerve root by a relatively rapidly placed high compression force (Fig 5–6, *top*). The result is intraneural injury, edema, inflammation, and the production of ectopic stimulus of pain. Stenosis, on the other hand, produces a slowly and circumferentially applied load. The root is irritated by motion in a tight canal, which causes edema, ischemia, and neurogenic claudication (Fig 5–6, *bottom*). The pain is aggravated by activity and relieved by rest. Neurogenic claudication may be unilateral (foramenal stenosis) or bilateral (central spinal canal stenosis). It can occur at any age and is associated with structural abnormalities in young patients (scoliosis or spondylolisthesis), and degenerative spondylolisthesis and/or ankylosing hyperostosis (Fournier's disease) in older patients.

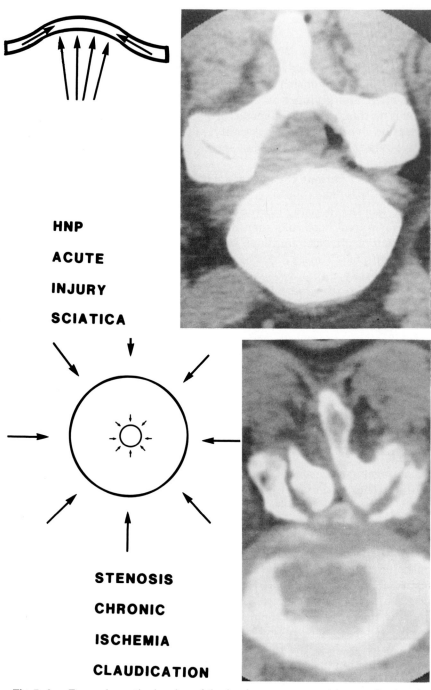

HNP

ACUTE

INJURY

SCIATICA

STENOSIS

CHRONIC

ISCHEMIA

CLAUDICATION

Fig 5–6.—*Top,* schematic drawing of the load on a nerve root from a disc hernia-tion and CAT scan showing large herniated disc displacing the S-1 nerve root and cauda equina. *Bottom,* schematic drawing depicting cross-section of nerve *(large circle)* and vasa nervorum *(small circle),* with circumferential forces *(large arrows)* causing ischemia *(small arrows).* Note the cauda equina squeezed into a small space on CAT scan with contrast.

CASE 3.—A 61-year-old male presented May 30, 1980, at University of Miami Hospital and Clinics with a 9-month history of back pain. The pain became worse with activity, was relieved by rest, localized to the back, and aggravated by extension. The patient had a negative neurovascular examination but tight hamstrings on straight leg raising at 70 degrees bilateral. Roentgenograms demonstrated degenerative spondylolisthesis at L4-5 with marked facet hypertrophy. At follow-up examinations, he consistently complained of mechanical back pain but no leg pain when walking. Stress films in June 1981 showed a 5-mm transla-

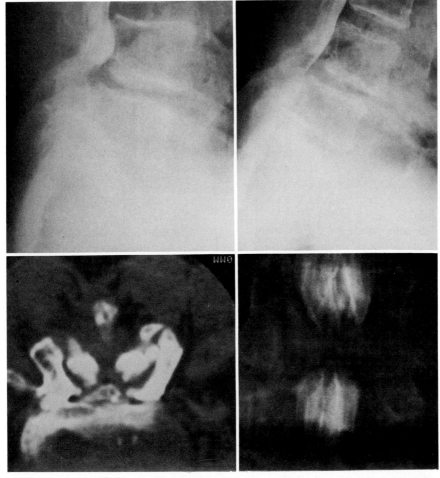

Fig 5–7.—*Top,* flexion and extension (lateral roentgenograms) with metrizamide myelogram, showing unstable degenerative spondylolisthesis with spinal stenosis and disc displacement at the L-4 lumbar interspace. *Bottom left,* computer-assisted tomogram with contrast, showing severe central spinal canal stenosis. *Bottom right,* anteroposterior metrizamide myelogram, showing high degree of blockage to flow of contrast at the L-4 lumbar interspace.

tion of the fourth vertebra on the fifth in the flexed position, which reduced to normal in the extended position. By April 1982, the patient had developed, over the previous 6 months, progressive bilateral leg pain made worse by walking and relieved by rest or flexing forward. In July 1982, a metrizamide myelogram and CAT scan (Fig 5–7) showed a high degree of contrast blockage secondary to spinal stenosis from degenerative spondylolisthesis and marked facet hypertrophy. Central disc displacement in extension was also evident. The patient's history was interesting in that he had a combination of mechanical back pain complaints and subsequently developed classic neurogenic claudication from central spinal canal stenosis. In August 1982, a decompression and fusion was performed at the L4-5 level. At 6-weeks follow-up, the patient was walking normally without leg pain. Neural compression had been caused by a gradual circumferential constriction of the cauda equina, which resulted in ischemia as a source of ectopic stimulus leading to bilateral leg pain. Mechanical back pain complaints were an important clue to mechanical insufficiency in this case. Chemonucleolysis would not have helped this patient by shrinking the anterior extradural defect and allowing more room in the spinal canal. We doubt if chemonucleolysis would have stimulated new collagen formation to stabilize the joint. Further disc narrowing in this case would have caused more severe compromise of the cauda equina. This patient is a classic example of one who should not be injected with an enzyme.

Symptomatic spinal stenosis is a contraindication to enzyme injection. It is therefore important to be able to differentiate the nerve root pain associated with this condition from radiculopathy pain caused by disc displacement.

VASCULAR CLAUDICATION

Leg pain that results from vasular insufficiency and resulting ischemia can be differentiated from neurogenic claudication by history. Patients with vascular claudication will be able to walk a short distance before extremity pain and loss of function forces them to stop. They then prefer to stand in place (to increase arterial perfusion pressure) rather than to sit. Vascular claudication is usually associated with diminished or absent peripheral pulses.[21]

Patients with spinal stenosis and neurogenic claudication would rather sit or flex the lumbar spine for relief when leg pain occurs from walking.

Abdominal pain, tenderness, bruits, and pulsatile masses, particularly in men over age 50, are clues to the diagnosis of a symptomatic abdominal aortic aneurysm. Occasionally, an impending rupture of an aneurysm may be preceded by low back pain. Chemonucleolysis should not be performed without first ruling out the presence of these vascular lesions. They should be treated first when they coexist with symptoms of disc disease.

DISC DISPLACEMENT

The diagnosis of disc displacement by physical examination was studied by Hudgins in 1970.[11] He showed that positive crossed straight leg raising was associated with a confirmed diagnosis of disc displacement at surgery in 97% of patients. Disc displacement at surgery was noted in 90% of patients with localized weakness, i.e., weak big toe extensor (Fig 5–8), indicative of fifth lumbar root involvement. Patients with asymmetric reflexes had a herniated disc found at surgery 90% of the time. Sensory deficit in a radicular distribution was least predictive of the physical findings, with only 70% of patients having a disc herniation confirmed at surgery (Table 5–3).

A sciatic list (scoliosis) (Fig 5–9), restriction of forward flexion of less than 20 degrees, straight leg raising positive at less than 50 degrees with pain below the knee increased by dorsiflexion of the foot (Fig 5–10), are highly predictive of lumbar radiculopathy from herniated disc. All follow-up studies have shown that patients who have any one or a combination of these objective findings have a better prognosis for invasive treatment, including chemonucleolysis with chymopapain.[4, 8, 22]

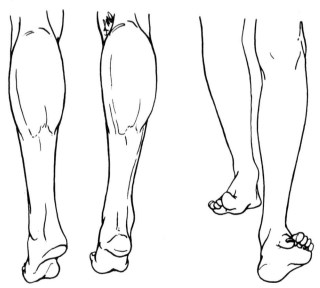

Fig 5–8.—Toe walking *(left)* and heel walking *(right)* give a clue to muscle weakness and localized lumbar radiculopathy. Note weak big toe extensor on the left foot, indicative of L-5 radiculopathy.

TABLE 5–3.—Preoperative
Physical Findings (%) in Patients
With Proved Disc Displacement

Painful crossed straight leg raising	97
Weakness	90
Asymmetric reflex	90
Sensory deficit	70
From Hudgins.[11]	

CONFIRMATION OF DIAGNOSIS

With the present state of the art, the diagnosis of a herniated disc must be confirmed by a good-quality metrizamide myelogram and/or computer assisted tomography (CAT scan).[23] We have injected patients whose herniated discs were confirmed by a positive high-resolution CAT scan alone. In these cases, the disc displacement noted on the CAT scan

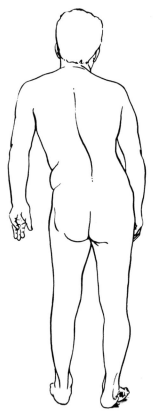

Fig 5–9.—Sciatic list of 20 degrees to the left in association with leg pain and positive straight leg raising gives a high degree of certainty to the diagnosis of lumbar radiculopathy from an extruded nucleus pulposus.

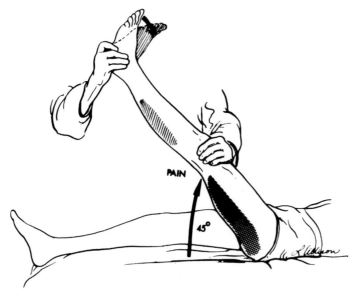

Fig 5–10.—Positive straight leg raising produces pain *(cross-hatched area)* in the sciatic nerve distribution at 45-degree elevation of the leg, extending to the calf by dorsiflexion of the foot *(hatched area).*

had to be at the level, and on the side of, objective physical findings of radiculopathy (see Fig 5–6). We realize that the rare coincidental tumor in the conus medullarus involving the same nerve root might be missed by not performing a myelogram and spinal fluid analysis. However, in the vast majority of patients, missing an extremely rare occurrence of a coincidental diagnosis of disc displacement and spinal cord tumor by depending on the confirmation of a CAT scan alone is more than justified by the avoidance of the risks of myelography. In all but the most straightforward cases in which a pain-producing herniated disc is suspected, we perform a metrizamide myelogram and CAT scan with the contrast still in place.[24]

Myelography

The myelogram enables the surgeon to see the entire subarachnoid space. Good visualization of the normal spinal cord, conus medullaris, lumbar roots, and nerve root sleeves can be obtained with metrizamide myelography. Coincidental nerve root anomalies, lateral recess, and central spinal canal stenosis coincidental with disc displacement can be found most easily by myelography. Multiple disc displacement is also easily recognized on the myelogram.

In patients who have already had surgery, the myelogram is imperative to rule out iatrogenic cyst and to help differentiate epidural scar tissue from herniated discs (Fig 5–11).

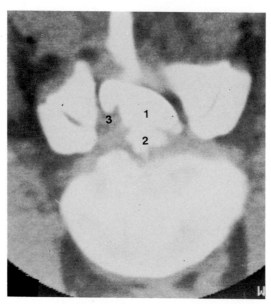

Fig 5–11.—Computer-assisted tomogram with contrast at the L-4 interspace in a patient with a third recurrent herniated nucleus pulposus at the same level on the same side. Metrizamide *(1)* in the distorted subarachnoid space can be distinguished from calcified herniated nucleus pulposus *(2)* from epidural scar *(3)* confirmed at surgery. We would not inject this patient.

A conus tumor or ependymoma may be detected by myelography and missed with other tests, including the CAT scan. Spinal fluid analysis should be correlated with myelography.

CAT Scan With Contrast

The CAT scan performed with partially diluted and absorbed contrast dye in the subarachnoid space imparts another dimension to diagnosis when one is trying to determine the exact source of pain. When disc displacement coincides with spinal stenosis and other spinal lesions, the CAT scan with contrast has been useful in determining whether chemonucleolysis will help relieve pain.

Epidural Venography and Discography

In rare instances, radiculopathy confirmed by history and physical examination cannot be demonstrated by a good-quality metrizamide myelogram and CAT scan. In such instances, confirmation by epidural venography[25] and/or discography[26] may be in order. We have not encountered such a case.

Spinal Fluid Analysis

A real advantage of performing the metrizamide myelogram before chemonucleolysis is that a spinal fluid sample can be obtained simultaneously. Adequate spinal fluid analysis, including cell count and differential as well as spinal fluid protein levels, should be obtained in all but the most straightforward cases of suspected herniated discs. In 186 disc displacement patients Hudgins found that the mean spinal fluid protein level was 35 mg%, with a range of 16–80 mg%. Compare these values to those in 11 patients with tumors who had a mean spinal fluid protein level of 173 mg% with a range of 50–570 mg%.[11]

Sequestrated Disc

Myelography also remains the most accurate method of examining the entire subarachnoid space to rule out development and/or acquired spinal stenosis, tumors, and sequestrated disc fragments (Fig 5–12), which contraindicate intradiscal enzyme injection. Occasionally, the myelogram shows an extradural defect over the silhouette of the vertebral body several centimeters away from the disc space (Fig 5–13). Using CAT scanning and carefully correlating the level of the transverse cuts, one can sometimes anticipate the existence of a sequestrated disc and thus avoid chemonucleolysis.

GENERAL RISKS

It is a mistake to assume that chemonucleolysis is an innocuous procedure and that high-risk patients—for example, cardiovascular cripples—should have this procedure because of its relative ease and safety compared with surgery. Chemonucleolysis has the small but ever-present risk of serious systemic allergic reaction which can be life threatening. The patient in marginal health, when exposed to this superimposed stress, would be placed at grave risk.

We have observed that the postinjection pain and stress following chemonucleolysis with either chymopapain or collagenase is greater than postoperative disc excision pain in most patients. Although Leavitt's comparison[27] using a multidimensional pain scale showed that the opposite was usually true, this has not been our experience.

PREINJECTION PATIENT PREPARATION

We make every effort to get people in proper condition before performing any invasive spinal procedure. For example, heavy smokers, drinkers, or medication abusers are detoxified before treatment.[28] Ridding the

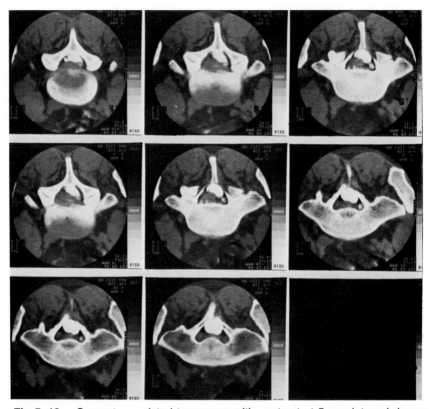

Fig 5–12.—Computer-assisted tomogram with contrast at 5-mm interval demonstrates a large extradural defect extending over 3.5 cm, bridging the entire L-5 vertebral body. A large sequestrated disc fragment was suspected and found at surgery. The patient was spared an enzyme injection.

body of 10% carboxyhemoglobin in heavy smokers and allowing the liver to rest in drinkers certainly seems justified before such patients are subjected to a stressful treatment regimen. Pretreatment detoxification has decreased the incidence of postsurgical morbidity in our patients. Also, if a serious allergic reaction occurs, the patient requires every physiologic advantage to survive.

One must be cautious with the patient who has been in bed for a prolonged period for a painful leg condition because these patients have a propensity to develop thromboembolic disease. Mobilization, hydration, and weaning from narcotic medication are indicated before any surgical procedure—and that most certainly includes chemonucleolysis—so that thromboembolic complications can be avoided or detected prior to invasive treatment (see Chap. 8).

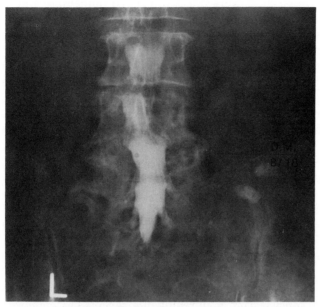

Fig 5–13.—Anteroposterior metrizamide myelogram, showing a large extradural defect bridging the entire fourth lumbar vertebral body on the right side in a 78-year-old man with severe leg pain that began one month before this study. A large sequestrated disc arising from the third lumbar interspace was suspected and confirmed at surgery.

REINJECTION

There are no contraindications to injecting collagenase into a patient who has previously been treated with chymopapain and vice versa. Some patients actually benefit from the two antigenically different intradiscal chemonucleolytic agents. If reherniation occurs, we do not anticipate contraindications to injecting the same disc that has been previously injected with the other agent. The reason for failure at the same disc level may be a failure of the agent to bind to the substrate, to be active, or to reach the offending disc material. Disc displacement probably recurs because of repeated trauma to fibrocartilage that formed in the interspace after the first injection. In either event, reinjection at the same level with a different agent should give the patient the same chance for satisfactory outcome as the first procedure.

CASE 4.—A 38-year-old male developed left sciatic pain following athletic activity in November 1969. In May 1980, a myelogram confirmed the diagnosis of disc displacement at L-5 on the left. The patient underwent chemonucleolysis with chymopapain in Toronto. Both the fourth and fifth lumbar discs were injected. He had immediate and lasting pain relief in the left leg until April 1982, when he developed recurrent left leg pain while riding on a tractor. In August 1982, a repeat myelogram demonstrated a large extradural defect on the left side at the fifth lumbar interspace. He was referred to the University of Miami Hospital and Clinics where, on physical examination, he had only 20 degrees of forward flexion, a positive straight leg raising at 30 degrees with pain into the calf, no left Achilles tendon reflex, a trace of weakness of the left extensor hallucis longus muscle and diminished sensation on the lateral aspect of the left foot. On September 1, 1982, the patient underwent chemonucleolysis at the fifth lumbar interspace with collagenase. He had immediate partial pain relief in the left leg, which gradually improved over the ensuing weeks. He returned to work within 4 days of the injection. Three months after injection, his excellent results continued. The availability of two antigenically different enzymes for chemonucleolysis benefited this patient, who was the first to be treated with both chymopapain and collagenase.

Reinjection with the same enzyme, however, is contraindicated because prior sensitization may result in a serious systemic reaction.

CONTRAINDICATIONS

Neurologic Deficit

Patients with major neurologic deficits should not be injected. Paralysis of the anterior tibial, extensor communis, and peroneal muscles resulting in complete foot drop constitutes one example of a major neurologic deficit. Another example is poor pushoff secondary to gastrocnemius-soleus muscle group paresis or paralysis (Fig 5–14). Bilateral motor weakness with severe bilateral leg pain with or without sphincter dysfunction and a large central disc herniation is a contraindication to disc injection (cauda equina syndrome secondary to disc prolapse).[29] Symptoms of a neurogenic bowel or bladder (e.g., urinary hesitancy or urgency, urinary retention, stress incontinence, loss of peroneal sensation and/or rectal tone, rectal incontinence) are contraindications to chemonucleolysis.

Usually, patients with the above symptoms and signs have a complete or nearly complete myelographic block secondary to a large disc displacement. In the absence of the above symptoms, such blocks or a large disc noted on CAT scan are relative contraindications to intradiscal injection.

CASE 5. (Fig 5–15).—A 32-year-old plumber complained of back and right leg pain that began in June 1982. The most recent pain episode

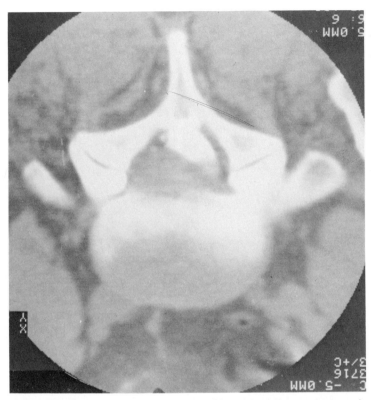

Fig 5–14.—Computer-assisted tomogram with contrast demonstrates a large extradural defect compromising more than half of the spinal canal. The patient had severe leg pain with paresis of the gastrocnemius and soleus muscles on the same side as the defect at the fifth lumbar interspace. Disc excision was followed by prompt relief of leg pain and return of pushoff.

was an exacerbation of chronic intermittent backache for many years. The patient had limited forward flexion, a scoliotic list of 10 degrees to the left, a positive straight leg raising on the right at 30 degrees with pain into the calf, and a contralateral positive straight leg raising on the left at 70 degrees with pain into the right thigh. There was hyperesthesia in S-1 distribution of the right foot and a trace of weakness of the right extensor hallucis longus muscle. The patient could not lie prone on the examining table because of marked increase in back and leg pain. A Pantopaque myelogram (Fig 5–15) demonstrated an apple-core constriction of a developmentally small spinal canal at the L5-S1 interspace. Chemonucleolysis is contraindicated in this case because there is no room for safe temporary expansion of the disc should this occur following injection. Furthermore, narrowing of this interspace would increase subluxation of the facet joint processes and possibly cause more posterior lateral spinal canal compromise.

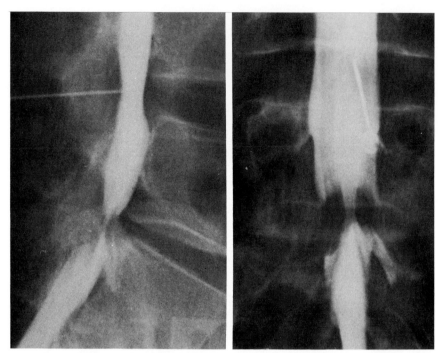

Fig 5–15.—Lateral *(left)* and anteroposterior *(right)* Pantopaque lumbar myelogram demonstrating a circumferential constriction of the dura at the fifth lumbar interspace, secondary to developmental stenosis and superimposed degenerative changes resulting in bulging of the annulus fibrosus and subluxation and hypertrophy of the facet joint process.

In these cases, we think that a major neurologic deficit following intradiscal injection may occur. Therefore, we recommend surgery with wide lateral exposure to remove the offending disc from the neural elements as the safe procedure in these cases. It must be pointed out, however, that two separate follow-up studies (Wiltse[30] and Javid[31]) have shown that chemonucleolysis with chymopapain is a gentle method of decompressing nerves compared to surgery, as shown by the higher percentage of reversal of neurologic deficit to normal following chemonucleolysis (see Table 2–3).

Pregnancy

At present, pregnancy or suspected pregnancy are contraindications to chemonucleolysis with either enzyme. The safety of this treatment during any phase of pregnancy remains to be determined in animal studies.

Previous Surgery

The indication for chemonucleolysis in patients who have undergone previous laminectomy and disc excision should be carefully determined by physicians experienced in evaluating and treating this difficult group of individuals. Repeated surgery for the relief of back pain has a prognosis that becomes progressively poorer with increasing numbers of procedures.[32, 33, 34]

The patient with a recurrent herniated disc at the same level who had a pain-free interval longer than 6 months, the patient with sciatic pain in the opposite extremity from that previously relieved by surgery, or the patient with sciatic pain resulting from a disc herniation at a level other than the one previously excised should respond to chemonucleolysis.

One must be careful when injecting a disc space previously exposed to surgery. It is difficult to determine whether an indolent disc space infection exists. One cannot be sure whether the dura has been compromised by surgery with subsequent adhesions, which would allow intradiscally injected substances to enter the subarachnoid space.

The most common reasons for failure of the first surgical procedure are unrecognized psychogenic regional pain disturbance, subsequent development of spinal stenosis, and/or foramenal entrapment. These conditions all respond poorly to chemonucleolysis.

REFERENCES

1. O'Connell J.E.A.: Protrusions of lumbar intervertebral discs: A clinical review based on 5000 cases treated by excision of the protrusion. *J. Bone Joint Surg.* 33B:8, 1951.
2. Hitselberger W.E., Witten R.M.: Abnormal myelograms in asymptomatic patients. *J. Neurosurg.* 28:204, 1968.
3. Pearce J., Moll J.M., II: Conservative treatment and natural history of acute lumbar disc lesions. *J. Neurol. Neurosurg. Psychiatry* 30:13, 1967.
4. Wiltse L.: Chemonucleolysis in ideal candidates for laminectomy. *The Spectator*, June 30, 1978.
5. Smith L.: Failures with chemonucleolysis. *Orthop. Clin. North Am.* 2:255, 1975.
6. Adams P., Eyre D., Muir H.: Biochemical aspects of development and aging of human lumbar intervertebral discs. *Rheumatol. Rehabil.* 16:22, 1977.
7. Nordby E.: Personal communication, August 1982.
8. Wiltse L.: Chemonucleolysis in ideal candidate for laminectomy. Personal communication, June 19, 1978.
9. Eyre D., Muir H.: Quantitative analysis of types I and II collagens in human intervertebral discs at various ages. *Acta Biochim Biphys.* 492:29, 1977.
10. Barrett A.J., Starkey P.M.: The interaction of α_2 macroglobulin with protease. *Biochem. J.* 133:709, 1973.
11. Hudgins P.W.: The predictive value of myelography in the diagnosis of ruptured lumbar discs. *J. Neurosurg.* 32:152, 1970.
12. Ransford A.D., Carrins C., Mooney V.: The pain drawing as an aid to the psychologic evaluation of patients with low back pain. *Spine* 1:127, 1976.

13. Murphy F.: Sources and patterns of pain in disc disease. *Clin. Neurosurg.* 15:343, 1968.

14. Brown M.D.: Low back strain and rupture of the intervertebral disc: section 2, Diagnosis of back pain syndromes; section 4, Treatment of painful back syndromes, in *Practice of Orthopaedic Surgery,* ed. 2. Hagerstown. Md., Harper & Row, 1977.

15. Brown M.D.: The diagnosis of back pain syndromes. *Orthop. Clin. North Am.* 6:233, 1975.

16. Brown M.D.: Lumbar spine fusion, in Finneson B.E. (ed.): *Low Back Pain,* ed. 2. Philadelphia, J.B. Lippincott Co., 1979.

17. Knutsson F.: The instability associated with disc degeneration in the lumbar spine. *Acta Radiol.* 25:593, 1944.

18. Wiltse L.L., Rocchio P.D.: Preoperative psychological tests as predictors of success of chemonucleolysis in the treatments of low back syndrome. *J. Bone Joint Surg.* 57A:478, 1975.

19. Waddell G., McCulloch J., Kummel E., Venny R.: Nonorganic physical signs in low back pain. *Spine* 5:11, 1980.

20. Grabias S.: The treatment of spinal stenosis. *J. Bone Joint Surg.* 42A:308, 1980.

21. Hawkes C.H., Roberts G.M.: Neurogenic and vascular claudication. *J. Neurol. Sci.* 38:337, 1978.

22. Spengler D.M., Freeman C.W.: Patient selection for lumbar discectomy. *Spine* 4:129, 1979.

23. Haughton V.M., Eldevik O.P., Magnaes B., Amerndsea P.: A prospective comparison of computed tomography and myelography in the diagnosis of herniated lumbar discs. *Radiology* 142:103, 1982.

24. Post M.J.D.: CT update: The impact of time, metrizamide, and high resolution on the diagnosis of spinal pathology, in Post M.J.D. (ed.): *Radiographic Evaluation of the Spine: Current Advances With Emphasis on Computer Tomography.* New York, Masson Publishers, 1980.

25. MacNab I., St. Louis E.L., Grabias S.L., Jacob R.: Selective ascending lumbosacral venography in the assessment of lumbar disc herniation. *J. Bone Joint Surg.* 58A:1093, 1976.

26. Abdulla A.F., Ditto E.W., Byrd E.W., Williams R.: Extreme lateral lumbar disc herniations. *J. Neurosurg.* 41:229, 1974.

27. Leavitt F., Garron D., Whisler W., et al.: A comparison of patients treated by chymopapain and laminectomy for low back pain using a multidimensional pain scale. *Clin. Orthop.* 146:136, 1980.

28. McLellon A.T., Lubrosky L., O'Brien C.P., et al.: Is treatment for substance abuse effective? *J.A.M.A.* 1423–1428, 1982.

29. Choudhury A.R., Taylor J.C.: Cauda equina syndrome in lumbar disc disease. *Acta Orthop. Scand.* 51:493, 1980.

30. Wiltse L.L., Widell E.H., Hansen A.Y.: Chymopapain chemonucleolysis in lumbar disc disease. *J.A.M.A.* 231:474, 1975.

31. Javid M.: Treatment of herniated lumbar disc syndrome with chymopapain. *J.A.M.A.* 243:2043, 1980.

32. Waddell G., Kummel E.G., Lotto W.N., et al.: Failed lumbar disc surgery and repeat surgery following industrial injuries. *J. Bone Joint Surg.* 61A:201, 1979.

33. Finnegan W.J., Fenlin J.M., Marvel J.P., et al.: Results of surgical intervention in the symptomatic multiply-operated back patient. *J. Bone Joint Surg.* 61A:1077, 1979.

34. Brown M.D.: Spinal Surgery: A Combined Neurosurgical and Orthopaedic Advanced Course. University of Miami School of Medicine, Miami Beach, Florida, April, 1982.

6 / Technique of Chemonucleolysis

THE OBJECTIVE of this technique is to deliver the enzyme to the offending disc material by a transcutaneous needle injection as simply and safely as possible without injuring adjacent structures (see Figs 5–1 and 5–2). The technique has evolved over the past 20 years to the point where it can be safely done on an outpatient basis with little anxiety, discomfort, and risk to the patient.[1] Patients have stated that the worst thing that happened to them by far was the myelogram during the course of diagnosis and disc injection. However, surgeons should not allow themselves to be lulled into complacency by the seeming simplicity of this procedure.

Among the early lessons that were learned in performing this technique was the risk of disc space infection as the result of penetrating the retroperitoneal space. Nerve root injury resulting in neurologic deficit or causalgia may have been caused by needle penetration of the neural structures.[2] Close attention to detail can eliminate these and other technical complications.

Most important, the surgeon must never forget the ever-present threat of an immediate, severe, life-threatening anaphylactic reaction.

If the indications and techniques of this procedure are thoroughly understood, we feel that this method is a real breakthrough in the management of disc displacement.

PHYSICAL FACILITIES

The major requirement for a location for chemonucleolysis is an area with adequate fluoroscopy to clearly visualize the disc space involved. Standby facilities for anesthesia with the appropriate resuscitative equipment must be available.

Whether chemonucleolysis is performed in the operating room or in the radiology department depends on individual circumstances. In our institution, we perform the procedure in the radiology department, in a fluoroscopy suite specifically designed for elective clean injection procedures. The Uniplaner fluoroscopy unit and table are quite versatile and provide a clear picture. There is adequate space for anesthesia equipment and room for easy access to the patient.

Our operating room staff and administrators are also delighted by the fact that we are not overburdening the operating theater with these procedures. Another advantage of performing the procedure in the radiology department is the rapidity and ease with which the staff can develop the films.

EQUIPMENT

The following items should be available for every chemonucleolysis procedure:

lead apron
fluoroscope
caps, gowns, masks
sterile gloves
prep and drape tray
marking pen
centimeter ruler
lidocaine 1%, 1 new vial
5-cc syringe with 18-gauge and 22-gauge needle for lidocaine
10-cc syringe with 18-gauge needle for Conray
Conray-60 (60% iothalamate), 1 new vial
3-cc syringes with 18 gauge needle for each disc to be injected
extension tubing with Leur-lok connections
4 6-inch 18-gauge needles with stylus
2 7-inch 22-gauge needles with stylus
lead-impregnated surgical gloves
radiation monitor badge

PATIENT PREPARATION

Preinjection Diagnosis

To avoid the compound effects, if any, of myelography and enzyme injection, we like an interval of at least 3 days between the myelogram and chemonucleolysis, if possible. Our patients are admitted as inpatients for 48 hours for a thorough history and physical examination, consultation with an internist and psychologist, laboratory studies, and myelography. We then discuss the diagnosis and the alternatives of care with the patient and the family before discharge and elective readmission at a later date. Any adverse reactions to the myelogram or psychological problems can thus be alleviated before any elective, invasive treatment program is begun. Information about the procedure (Fig 6–1) and an informed consent form (Fig 6–2) are also given at this time.

The patient is now ready to be treated as an outpatient. He or she can be seen in the ambulatory care unit in the morning, injected, observed for 2 hours, and allowed to go home. Outpatient chemonucleolysis

Your doctor has diagnosed your condition as a herniated (slipped) disc in the low back, causing your back pain and/or leg pain.

Treating your herniated disc by enzyme injection has a major advantage of avoiding surgery and the accompanying risks. The purpose of the injection is to chemically dissolve or shrink that part of the disc that is causing pressure on the nerve and pain in your leg. Following injection therapy, you have between a 70 and 85% chance of a good or excellent result, with complete relief of leg pain and return to your full work and recreational activity. No further treatment should be required.

Patients who have injections have a variable course for the first 4 to 6 weeks. Some patients get dramatic and immediate relief of leg pain with a slight recurrence between 10 days and 2 weeks after injection. Some patients are able to return to work as soon as 2 weeks after injection, but those that do heavy work and lifting require at least 6 weeks and sometimes longer before returning to work. Other patients have a marked increase in back pain, which lasts between 3 and 6 weeks before they obtain final relief. We do not know why some patients have more pain than others with this procedure.

The injection treatment to dissolve your disc requires you to be in the hospital for at least one day. You will be admitted the night before or, in some cases, the morning of the procedure. You should not eat or drink anything after midnight of the night before the procedure. Scrub your back with soap for 10 minutes the night before the procedure.

Just before the procedure, an intravenous line will be placed in the arm on the same side as your leg pain. You will be given injections of medication to prevent or decrease the severity of an allergic reaction to the enzyme, should it occur. Then you will be taken to the x-ray department on a stretcher.

In x-ray, you will lie on your side and an anesthesiologist will be in attendance. The anesthesiologist will give you a pain killer and a tranquilizer so that you will be slightly sedated and yet will be able to cooperate with the doctor during the procedure. The doctor will prepare your back and your side with a cold antiseptic solution. He will then inject the skin with a local anesthetic to numb it so that you will not have pain from the needle insertion. Most patients say that they have less pain and anxiety from this injection than they do from a myelogram. The needle is inserted through the numbed skin into the disc. Fluoroscopy helps the surgeon place the needle properly into the disc. X-rays are then taken as a permanent record of which disc was injected and of the adequacy of the needle placement. During this procedure you are exposed to a small dose of x-ray from fluoroscopy. X-ray contrast dye will then be injected into the disc to confirm the diagnosis and help your doctor decide how much enzyme to inject to dissolve the disc. More permanent x-rays will be taken, and some time will go by before the enzyme will be injected. After the dye has been injected, you may feel increased back pain and/or leg pain like that which you have been suffering before the injection. If at any time during the procedure you should feel pain radiating below the knee or into your foot, tell the doctor. Also, if you want to stop at any time during this procedure, all you have to do is tell the doctor. We have found that even the most frightened patients have found the procedure to be nonthreatening and quite tolerable. The entire procedure takes 20-60 minutes.

The enzyme will then be injected. You have less than a 1% chance of having an allergic reaction to the chemical. If this should happen, you may experience itching, a tingling sensation, wheezing, nausea, or vomiting. If these symptoms occur, inform the doctor immediately. The doctor and the anesthesiologist are fully trained and know how to treat an allergic reaction. The chance of a severe allergic reaction requiring intensive treatment is about one in 200 injections. Unfortunately, there is no method available today to determine who will be allergic and who will not. However, if you are allergic to papaya fruit, meat tenderizer, or have already had a chymopapain injection into your disc(s), you should inform your doctor, and not have chymopapain enzyme. If you have been treated with collagenase burn ointment (brand name _____)inform your doctor, and you should not have collagenase enzyme.

Most patients experience a short period of increased back pain just after injection of the enzyme. Some patients have noted dramatic decrease in their leg pain within minutes after the injection. You will be observed in the x-ray room for approximately half an hour and then go to the recovery room for an additional hour. Then you will be taken back to your hospital room or be observed in the ambulatory care center until all of the effects of the sedation and medication have worn off and you are able to walk and void. You will be discharged the same day or the following morning.

The doctor will see you in the outpatient clinic 2 weeks after injection, then 6 weeks, 3 months, and a year after injection. If you need to be seen at any other time or have any questions, feel free to call your doctor. This is important so that you do not worry about symptoms that you might experience. Most patients have some back and leg pain off and on for 4 to 6 weeks after injection. It should gradually subside. If you have not started to improve between 4 and 6 weeks after the injection, you may require surgery.

We have found that some patients require a corset, particularly in the first 2 weeks. About one-third of the patients injected have pain severe enough to require medication. We ask you to use as little pain medication as possible and to be as active as the pain permits. Try to stay in optimum health by avoiding drugs, alcohol, and tobacco. Exercise regularly as soon as pain permits. Swimming under supervision and walking are the best exercises for the first 6 weeks.

If you have any questions about the procedure write them down, so that you can remember to ask them.

Fig 6–1.—Preinjection instructions for patients.

SUGGESTED INFORMED CONSENT

BENEFIT OF PROCEDURE

For an extended period of time you have had back pain and leg pain which has been diagnosed as having been caused by a herniated disc. You have been advised that further conservative care may require several months without assurance of relief of pain. You have also been advised that you are an ideal candidate for a surgical disc excision.

You have been advised that a reasonable alternative to surgery is to have your disc chemically dissolved with the enzyme _____. When this enzyme is injected into the disc space it should cause the disc to dissolve gradually over a four to six week period and relieve the pressure on the nerve thus relieving the leg pain. More than 70% of patients can expect to have satisfactory relief of symptoms. In those patients in whom the drug does not work the chance of relief from subsequent surgery is not compromised.

NATURE OF THE PROCEDURE

The procedure will involve placing needle(s) into the herniated disc(s) to inject the enzyme into the disc. This will be done in x-ray, using fluoroscopy (x-ray television) to monitor the needle placement. Prior to the injection you will be temporarily numbed with a local anesthetic agent. You will be awake for the procedure which takes between 20 and 60 minutes. During the procedure, intravenous fluids will be running into your vein and an anesthesiologist will be present in order that you may receive prompt treatment should a reaction occur.

Following the procedure, you will be observed in the recovery room for approximately an hour and then will be allowed to walk with assistance the first time. Most patients experience increase back and/or leg pain following injection which may last as long as two weeks. This means the enzyme is working.

POSSIBLE RISKS

Fewer than one patient in one hundred who receive an enzyme injection experience an adverse reaction. Rarely a severe allergic reaction requiring immediate treatment by the doctor and anesthesiologist has occurred following enzyme injection. With the proper treatment, promptly performed, the risk of this reaction causing death or permanent damage is very low. There have been rare cases of paralysis, numbness, bleeding, infection, nerve damage, increased pain, bowel or bladder disturbance, allergic reactions and death or other side effects occurring as the result of enzyme treatment. However, comparing the risks of this treatment to the risks of surgery showed that it is five times safer than surgery. Either surgical treatment or enzyme treatment is very safe and risks are small.

There is a chance that the procedure cannot be completed safely once started because of technical difficulties or diagnostic findings on the discogram.

Fig 6–2.—Suggested patient consent form.

should only be done when the patient has immediate access to the physician and the inpatient facility, should an adverse reaction occur. The most common problem encountered in the first 10 days after injection is increased pain and anxiety, which can be handled by immediate telephone access to the doctor for reassurance.

Preinjection Preparation

The night before the injection, we ask patients to shower with an antiseptic soap and scrub the back and flank on the side of the leg pain for 10 minutes. The same procedure is repeated on the morning of the injection. The patient should not eat or drink after midnight the night before the procedure. The morning of the procedure, an intravenous line with a large (18-gauge) catheter is inserted in the arm on the side of the leg pain. The line is kept open with a small bottle of 5% dextrose in water (50 ml/hr or less). On call to the radiology department, at least 30 minutes before the procedure, the patient is given diphenhydramine (Benadryl) 100 mg intramuscularly and hydrocortisone (Solu-Cortef) 100 mg intramuscularly.[3] The patient is then asked to void and is sent to the radiology department on a stretcher.

POSITION FOR FLUOROSCOPY

We perform the procedure by inserting the needle in the same side as the symptomatic leg pain (Fig 6–3). Patients with left-side sciatica are placed in the right lateral decubitus position on the fluoroscopy table, and the needle is inserted on the left side. The objective is to place the tip of the needle within the disc space as close to the point of disc herniation as possible so that on discography the extradural defect previously noted on the myelogram and/or CAT scan is infiltrated by the contrast dye. We can then assume that the subsequently injected enzyme will reach the offending disc material (Plates 2 and 3).[4] A well-

Fig 6–3.—Diagram of a patient in the right decubitus position, showing angles of needle insertion by the lateral approach into the lumbosacral disc. Insertion begins 11 cm lateral to the L4-5 interspace and just above the iliac crest, with the needle 30 degrees caudad and at a 45-degree angle to the sagittal plane. Patient has left-side sciatica.

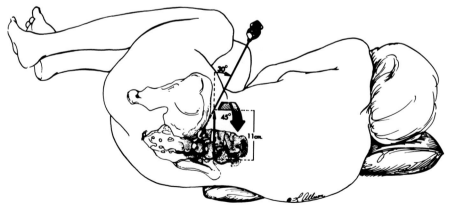

placed needle and positive confirming discogram can be performed from either the right or left side. The choice of side(s) to be injected is up to the surgeon.

We prefer the lateral decubitus position for ease of visualization of the disc space on the Uniplaner fluoroscope. By altering the height of a small towel roll placed under the recumbent flank, one can get a true lateral fluoroscopic view of the disc, especially the fifth lumbar disc space. Also, by altering the flexion of the hips and knees, one can change the angle of obstruction of the posterior iliac crest for easier access to the fifth lumbar disc. It is easy for the patient to cooperate by rotating the nonrecumbent hemipelvis toward or away from the surgeon a few millimeters for a pure lateral fluoroscopic view of the disc. In case of a systemic reaction requiring immediate treatment, the patient can be turned rapidly and easily to a supine position.

Some surgeons prefer the prone position for this procedure.[5] They state that it is very easy on the patient and that the extension of the hips rotates the ilium and lumbosacral spine into a lordotic position, which facilitates entry into the lumbosacral disc.

The prone position requires adequate biplane fluoroscopy or a C-arm that can be rotated and a Collis table.[6] It would take longer to rotate the patient to the supine position should a systemic reaction occur. Intra-abdominal pressure is increased and the viscera forced posteriorly against the retroperitoneum.

Whether the prone position has any advantage in avoiding needle penetration of the retroperitoneal space has not been determined. Surgeons become accustomed to performing tasks in the way that they were taught. In this regard, I was taught needle insertion with the patient in the lateral decubitus position, and I prefer it for the reasons stated above. I also can clearly visualize the three-dimensional spatial relationships by this approach.

ANESTHESIA

The preferred analgesic for chemonucleolysis is lidocaine 1% injected locally into the skin and lumbar fascia. An anesthesiologist should be in attendance to monitor the patient's blood pressure and heart beat. Analgesia is supplemented by administrating intravenous diazepam, 3–5 mg and/or fentanyl, 50–150 μg. Occasionally, we supplement these medications with 60% N_2O mixed with 40% O_2. We like the patient to have maximum amnesia and analgesia, but at the same time to be cooperative enough to flex and extend the hips slightly or to rotate the pelvis. We also want the patient to be able to inform us of leg pain radiating below the knee secondary to needle penetration of the nerve root or sensory ganglia (Plate 4). We avoid general anesthesia because the patient would not be able to inform us of this potential complication.

The other major reason for local anesthesia is that we like the patient to be able to cooperate and inform us of any immediate postinjection symptoms that would help us recognize the early onset of anaphylactic reaction. The existing theory is that the earlier the recognition of these reactions and the earlier the injection of epinephrine, the better the chance of avoiding severe progressive changes.[7] If general anesthesia is used, avoid halothane, which increases cardiac excitability that could become a problem if subsequent administration of adrenaline is required. Also the use of curare as a muscle relaxant should be avoided because it releases histamine, one of the medications for anaphylaxis.[8]

LOCALIZATION

With a marking pen, indicate the location of the iliac crest and the posterior superior iliac spine, which are found by palpation. Also, palpate the center of the spinous processes and mark it. Using a ruler, make a mark just superior to the posterior superior iliac spine and iliac crest 10 cm lateral to the tip of spinous process of the third lumbar vertebra (Fig 6–4). Next, prepare the skin with Betadine and drape with sterile towels. Between 8 and 10 cm lateral to the third lumbar spinous process and just superior to the iliac spine, where the mark has previously been made, infiltrate the subcutaneous tissue with 2 ml of 1% lidocaine.

To gain the patient's confidence and alleviate anxiety, be constantly gentle; tell him everything that you are about to do—including palpation, marking the skin, prepping with cold antiseptic solution, and the painful subcutaneous injection of local anesthetic. If these steps are taken first, the patient will require less analgesic medication and will be more cooperative and less anxious.

CHOICE OF NEEDLES

We now use 6-inch, 18-gauge needles with a stylus almost exclusively. We have available an 8-inch, 22-gauge needle that fits through the 18-gauge needle for rare cases when it is difficult to penetrate the lumbo-·sacral disc space due to narrowing. The 18-gauge needle is just stiff enough not to bend easily when penetrating the various tissues. The bevel on the end is large enough to act like the rudder of a ship. By rotating the needle so that the bevel faces away from the area toward which you want to direct the needle, you can steer the needle through the tissue planes. On the hub of the stylus and needle is an interlocking mechanism that is always on the same side as the bevel of the needle. Therefore, you can always tell the orientation of the bevel by the notch at the hub (Plate 5).

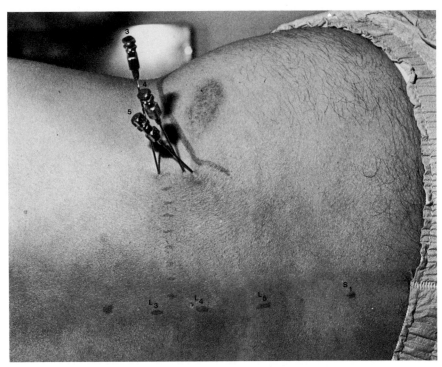

Fig 6–4.—Posterior view of points of needle insertion into the third, fourth, and fifth lumbar discs in a patient with a transitional fifth lumbar vertebra. The needles are numbered according to the discs in which they are inserted. The tips of the spinous processes and the iliac crest have been marked, and centimeter marks have been made lateral to the interspinous ligament between the third and fourth spinous processes.

NEEDLE PLACEMENT AND INSERTION

After donning a lead apron with a gown, mask, hood, and two pairs of surgical gloves, insert the needle at the previous spot between 8 and 11 cm lateral to the midline. To enter the lumbosacral disc space, which is the most difficult to penetrate, insert the needle at an angle of 45 degrees to the sagittal plane of the body and 30 degrees to the transverse plane, until the needle is stable without being held and a fluoroscopic view can be obtained. Make sure that the orientation of the spine with respect to superior, inferior, anterior, and posterior on the fluoroscopy screen is the same as the anatomical orientation of the patient on the table. The fluoroscopist can switch the image backward and forward or superior and inferior to meet your orientation requirements. Initially, the fluoroscopist should show you the disc space that you want to inject in relation to the tip of the needle and the angle of the needle shaft. Use as little fluoroscopy as possible to gain a mental image of these relationships. With experience, it requires less than 12 seconds of fluoroscopy per patient.[9] We recommend that the surgeons who perform these procedures wear an x-ray monitor badge to ensure that they do not exceed recommended safety levels for radiation exposure.

Next, correct the angulation of the needle and insert it to the level of the pars interarticularis (Plate 6). Have another look at the fluoroscope. If continued insertion of the needle along the same angulation will bring the tip to the superior posterolateral corner of the disc space, continue the injection. The bevel at this time should be facing directly laterally so that the needle tip tends to keep the needle snug against the superior facet process of the vertebra on which the disc to be injected rests, that is, the fifth lumbar superior facet for the fourth lumbar disc. If the bevel is pointed superiorly or inferiorly, the needle will tend to be directed inferiorly or superiorly, respectively. If the facet joint capsule is irritated by penetration of the needle tip, the patient will experience localized back pain and/or referral into the buttocks or trochanteric region but not below the knee. If the angle of insertion is not correct, as determined by fluoroscopy, withdraw the needle until it is no more than 3–5 cm into the muscle and then redirect it properly before reinserting. If the needle is withdrawn completely, use a new needle to avoid multiple skin punctures with the same needle. Try to keep a mental image from the short fluoroscopic exposure (how many degrees angulation change, in what direction the change should be) before withdrawing the needle and reinserting it. Once the needle is more than 5 cm into the body, it is difficult to change direction by correcting angulation. When the tip of the needle has reached the depth of the facet joints and pars interarticularis, and the angulation and direction are correct, advance the needle a centimeter at a time and spot-check by fluoroscopy. When it has reached the posterolateral and superior corner of the disc to be injected, you should feel a rubbery resistance. Between the pars interarticularis and posterolateral corner of the disc, 1 cm advancement of the needle itself should correspond to half a centimeter advance on the fluoroscope, if the angulation is correct (Plate 6). One centimeter advancement of the needle with no advancement on fluoroscopy means the angle of insertion is too large with respect to the sagittal plane of the body and the needle will enter the spinal canal and penetrate the dura. If, on inserting the needle one centimeter, you notice advancement of one centimeter on fluoroscopy, the angle of insertion is too small with respect to the sagittal plane of the body. Continued insertion of the needle at this angle will penetrate the retroperitoneum.

If the patient complains of acute severe pain radiating below the knee while the needle is inserted between the depth of the facet joints and the posterolateral corner of the disc, a nerve root has been penetrated.

The needle should be withdrawn and a new one reinserted 1 cm distal to the original starting point, but at the same angle and direction as the first needle.

When the needle touches the posterolateral corner of the disc, the patient may experience localized back pain or radiation into the buttocks. This is particularly true with a sensitive peripheral annulus fibrosus inflamed by a herniated disc.[10] If a rubbery resistance is felt, the needle can be inserted into the disc. Advance the needle about 2 cm and spot-check by fluoroscopy. Before advancing the needle, particularly in the lumbosacral disc, due to the acute angle of approach to the disc to clear the iliac crest, it may be necessary to rotate the needle so that the bevel faces inferiorly in order to steer the needle around the corner of the vertebra (Plate 5). The needle will actually bend around the corner of the vertebra and into the center of the disc from the posterolateral corner.

Occasionally, it is difficult to insert an 18-gauge needle directly into the lumbosacral disc because the angle of approach is too acute. This situation usually occurs when there is narrowing in the two lower lumbar discs. The disc narrowing itself, in conjunction with the fifth vertebra settling farther below the iliac crest, increases the angle of lateral approach. When this happens, we use a two-needle technique. After the 18-gauge needle with stylus is injected to the level of the superior lateral corner of the disc, withdraw the stylus and insert a 22-gauge 8-inch needle with stylus, which has been previously curved at the end (3 cm). Penetrate the L5-S1 disc with the precurved 22-gauge needle (Plate 7).

Once the needle tip is in the nucleus pulposus in the central portion of the disc, the bevel can be turned superiorly. A large lateral x-ray and an anteroposterior x-ray are taken. On the AP view, a line is drawn through the tips of the spinous processes (Fig 6–5). The tip of the needle should be on this line. Note that the disc space at the lumbosacral end is seldom seen on the routine AP view, due to the forward inclination, 15–30 degrees, of the lumbosacral disc. On the lateral view, an imaginary line is drawn through the center of the vertebral bodies and sacrum (Fig 6–6), and the tip of the needle should lie on this line. The AP and lateral plain x-rays are a permanent record of the insertion level and the central placement of the needle tip in the disc to be injected.

DISCOGRAPHY

A 5-ml syringe and extension tubing filled with 60% iothalamate (Conray-60) are then attached to the hub of the needle after removing the stylus. While monitoring with fluoroscopy, inject Conray-60; avoid exposure to the hands by using the extension tubing. Leur-lok tubing helps to prevent explosion of the contrast because of the tubing slipping off the hub.

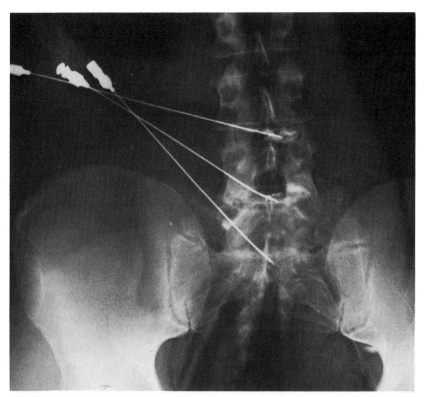

Fig 6–5.—Anteroposterior roentgenogram after needle insertion in patient shown in Figure 6–4. Tips of the needles are in line with the spinous processes in the center of the discs. The lumbosacral disc space is not visible in this projection, due to its forward inclination. The caudal angle of insertion into the disc was more acute than usual, due to the large transverse process at this level.

Several observations should be made at discography. The first is the resistance to injection. A severely degenerated disc that leaks has no resistance to injection. Don't inject more dye than is necessary to establish the diagnosis. An intact herniated disc will have moderate resistance, and a normal disc will have a very high resistance with little flow of contrast (less then 0.5 ml). Injecting a normal disc should rarely be necessary if adequate prescreening has been done. If a normal discogram pattern appears, do not force the dye in because this may cause pressure necrosis in the cells of the nucleus pulposus and subsequent discitis (Fig 6–7,a). In the herniated disc, try to inject enough dye to fill the area that corresponds to the extradural defect on myelography or CAT scan (Fig 6–7,b). The patient may complain of reproduction of the usual leg pain at this point. If the dye leaks into the epidural space, stop injecting (Fig 6–7,c). An epidural leakage of dye occurs in 15%–25% of discs injected, and is not a contraindication to chemonucleolysis.

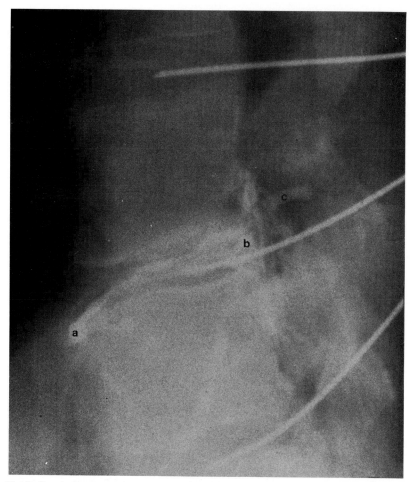

Fig 6–6.—Lateral roentgenogram after injection of contrast dye; same patient as Figure 6–4. Needle tips are in the centers of the discs. Contrast flowed into an anterior annulus defect at a lower pressure (a) than the dye flow into the posterior annulus defect (b). Note the avascular channel fills from the posterior defect (c).

However, if the contrast runs from the disc space into the subdural or subarachnoid space and causes bilateral severe leg pain, suspect an intradural herniation. This is a rare occurrence but has been estimated to happen in one in seven hundred cases of disc displacement.[11] If this situation is suspected, neither chymopapain or collagenase should be injected; and the procedure should be abandoned.

Fifteen of one hundred discs studied by cinefluoroscopy discography performed on unfixed cadaver lumbar spines demonstrated an immediate flow of contrast from the intradiscal space into a subchondral vascular channel or into a vascular channel in the peripheral layers of the annulus fibrosus in a degenerated herniated disc.[12] We have observed

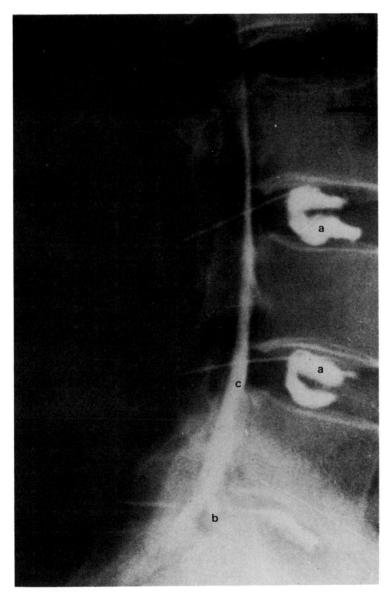

Fig 6–7.—Lateral roentgenogram showing a normal discogram pattern at the third and fourth lumbar interspace *(a)*, a posterior protrusion *(b)*, and an epidural leakage of dye *(c)*.

rapid intravascular flow of x-ray contrast dye at discography and before chemonucleolysis. This phenomenon is a relative contraindication to subsequent enzyme injection. The rapid flow of dye into the intravascular space at a low pressure would mean that a subsequent injection would take the same path and probably would not reach the offending disc herniation. A rapid intravascular injection of enzyme may contribute to the severity of an allergic reaction, should it occur.

Note the volume of injected contrast dye, in order to estimate the volume of enzyme to be injected. If there is an epidural leakage of contrast, inject the enzyme in increments over a long period of time, 5–10 minutes, so that the enzyme flows slowly into the disc and has time to bind to the disc matrix substance. Anteroposterior and lateral plain x-rays may then be taken as a permanent record. Wait approximately 15 minutes before injecting the enzyme in order to rule out an allergic reaction to the contrast dye. It has recently been shown in a very careful study by Naylor and associates that x-ray contrast dye does not inhibit the action of chymopapain on nucleus pulposus.[13] Recent collagenase studies in our laboratories have yielded evidence that the same is true for this enzyme (see Chap. 8).

To inject the fourth lumbar disc, insert the needle adjacent to the same insertion point for the lumbosacral disc. Begin between 8 and 11 cm lateral to the point between the fourth and fifth spinous process. Point the bevel laterally, and the stylus is in place. Insert an 18-gauge 6-inch needle far enough into the paraspinal muscle at an angle of 45 degrees to the sagittal plane until the needle is stationary when not held. Check fluoroscopically to determine if the angle of insertion in relation to the disc space is correct. Take care again to advance the needle slowly when the tip has reached the level of the facet joint. The first through fourth lumbar intervertebral discs are easily entered posterolaterally with a little practice.

We frequently refer to an articulated skeleton before doing this procedure to review the special relationships of the discs to the facet joints and the iliac crest.

ENZYME INJECTION

Chymopapain is supplied in a lyophilized 20-mg vial containing 10,000 units and stored at −10 C. The enzyme is reconstituted with sterile water without additives. Five milliliters of sterile water are injected into the vial, and the contents are slowly dissolved in the water by rotating the vial gently. The vial should not be shaken, and bubbles should not form. The resulting mixture contains 4 mg (2,000 units) per milliliter of chymopapain. Between 4 and 12 mg, 1–3 ml, of this mixture are injected into each disc space. A further precaution of interposing a Milex filter between the syringe and needle hub to ensure sterility of the enzyme may be taken. This should not be necessary, however, because the enzyme is supplied in a sterile vial. Injection should be made slowly and smoothly to allow adequate flow and binding of the chymopapain to the substrate. The anesthesiologist should be alert, and the patient should be cooperative enough to inform you of any symptoms of systemic allergic reaction. The blood pressure is taken at 1-minute intervals for the next 5 minutes, at 2-minute intervals for the next 10 minutes, and at 5-minute intervals for the next 15 minutes. Thirty minutes after injection, the patient should be taken to the recovery room by the anesthesiologist and the surgeon. We keep 10 ml of a 1:10,000 dilution of epinephrine in a labeled syringe taped to the front of the patient's chart. The patient is observed for another 30 to 60 minutes in the recovery room, after which he is returned to his room. In outpatient chemonucleolysis, the patient should be observed until all the effects of analgesics and sedatives have subsided; he should then be taken home by a relative or friend.

Collagenase is supplied in a vial containing slightly more than 1 ml of frozen enzyme suspension and should be stored between -15 C and -20 C. Special instructions concerning dilution of the enzyme to the final solution containing 600 units of collagenase per milliliter come with each batch of vials. Between 300 and 600 units are injected per disc. At present, no more than two discs per patient should be injected, i.e., 1,200 units per patient.

MANAGEMENT OF IMMEDIATE SYSTEMIC ALLERGIC REACTION

The pathophysiology of immediate systemic allergic reaction is reviewed in Chapter 7. Management of anaphylaxis is the same, despite the antigen that initiates the reaction. A prior knowledge of the incidence and risk involved with chymopapain allows the surgeon to prevent some cases of allergic reaction by eliminating patients who have a history of allergy to papaya fruit, meat tenderizer containing papain, or a history of prior injection with chymopapain. Chymopapain may have a slightly higher propensity for inducing an immediate systemic allergic reaction than do other drugs. For this reason, prevention may include avoiding injection of patients who have a highly allergic history. In anticipation of these reactions, the patient should be premedicated with diphenhydramine, 50–100 mg and hydrocortisone, 100 mg intramuscularly within the hour before enzyme injection.

Anticipation of a reaction is essential. Have the patient optimally prepared, under local anesthesia for early recognition, a large intravenous catheter in place, anesthesia standby with light sedation, a cardiac monitor in place and running, and the team prepared for early treatment.

Early recognition of the reaction is of paramount importance. There is some evidence that immediate recognition of the reaction and immediate administration of epinephrine and large volumes of intravenous fluids may alter the outcome by preventing catastrophic deterioration of the patient.

If the patient becomes anxious or develops tingling, itching, paresthesia, "gooseflesh," hives, flush, wheezing, or stridor, in any combination, begin treatment immediately. It is possible that the patient may not have any cutaneous or respiratory symptoms but may present with hypotension,[14] arrhythmias, loss of consciousness, or severe cardiovascular collapse. Increase the flow of intravenous fluids, administer 1–3 ml of a 1:10,000 solution of epinephrine intramuscularly or intravenously, depending on the severity of the reaction, and turn the patient supine. Monitor the blood pressure every minute. If it does *not* respond to epinephrine, increase the flow of intravenous fluids and, if the patient has not developed a cardiac arrhythmia, administer additional epinephrine intravenously. If the patient develops wheezing and dyspnea that does not respond to epinephrine, administer aminophylline, 250 mg in 500 cc of solution over 15 minutes. Severe stridor as a result of laryngeal edema and dyspnea should be managed by an endotracheal tube which, if impossible to insert, should be replaced by tracheotomy.

As hypotension responds to epinephrine and intravenous fluid, additional diphenhydramine, 50–100 mg and hydrocortisone, 100–200 mg intravenously are indicated. When the patient's condition has been stabilized for at least 30 minutes, he may be taken to the recovery room. If he remains unstable, he should be transferred to an intensive care unit.

FOLLOW-UP CARE

After release from the recovery room following an hour of observation, the patient may walk with assistance. He should be able to walk and void spontaneously without difficulty before being allowed to go home. The neurologic examination should not show any findings worse than before the injection. If the patient is to remain in the hospital, the intravenous line may be discontinued and the preinjection diet resumed. Appropriate oral analgesics and sedatives are ordered as necessary.

REFERENCES

1. McCulloch J., Ferguson J.: Outpatient chemonucleolysis. *Spine* 6:606, 1981.
2. Watts C.: Complications of chemonucleolysis for lumbar disc disease. *Neurosurgery* 1:2, 1977.
3. Kelly J., Patterson R., Luberman P., et al.: Radiographic contrast media studies in high risk patients. *J. Allergy Clin. Immunol.* 62:181, 1978.
4. Brown M.D.: Chemonucleolysis with Discase: Technique, results, case reports. *Spine* 1:115, 1976. Erratum, 1:116, 1976.
5. Bromley J.: Personal communication, August 1982.
6. Collis J.S., Gardiner W.J.: Lumbar discography: An analysis of one thousand cases. *J. Neurosurg.* 19:452, 1962.
7. Kelly J., Patterson R.: Anaphylaxis: Course, mechanism and treatment. *J.A.M.A.* 227:1431, 1974.
8. Rajagopalan R., Tindal S., MacNab I.: Anaphylactic reactions to chymopapain during general anesthesia: A case report. *Anesth. Analg.* 53:191, 1974.
9. McCulloch J.A.: Personal communication, August 1982.

10. Smyth M.J., Wright, W.W.: Sciatica and the intervertebral disc. *J. Bone Joint Surg.* 40A:1401, 1958.
11. Blikra G.: Intradural herniated lumbar disc. *J. Neurosurg.* 31:676, 1969.
12. Lindahl S., Brown M., Irstam L., et al.: Roentgenologic Grading of Disc Degeneration by Discography. Paper presented to International Society for the Study of the Lumbar Spine, Toronto, 1982.
13. Naylor A., Earland C., Robinson J.: The effect of diagnostic radio-opaque fluids used in discography on chymopapain activity. *Spine,* accepted for publication, 1983.
14. McCulloch J.A.: Personal communication, August 1982.

7 / Failures and Complications of Chemonucleolysis

FAILURES WITH chemonucleolysis occur in 7%–30% of the cases treated,[1, 2] depending on the care taken in patient selection and attention to details of the technique. The average failure rate in our clinic is 15%. Eight of 49 patients whom we have managed by chymopapain injection failed to obtain relief and have required surgery. Three patients of the first 20 whom we treated with intradiscal collagenase injections have required surgery, and one patient has failed to obtain the desired result.

FAILURE TO RELIEVE SCIATICA

There are several reasons why an enzyme will fail to dissolve the displaced disc and relieve pressure on the neural elements. The first of these is failure of the enzyme to reach the offending disc material. The patient may have a sequestrated fragment of disc in the spinal canal that cannot imbibe the intradiscally injected enzyme (Plates 8 and 9).

CASE 1.—Thirty-seven-year-old male had insidious onset of right leg pain over 3 months. He had a 17-year history of intermittent back pain, which seemed to clear up when the leg pain began. He had had no relief, despite 10 days of hospitalization with bedrest and traction. A myelogram demonstrated a large extradural defect lateral at the fifth lumbar interspace consistent with disc displacement. On first examination at the University of Miami Hospital and Clinics in May 1982, the patient had limited forward flexion to 30 degrees, a positive straight leg raising on the right at 20 degrees with pain referral into the calf, a positive cross straight leg raising of the left leg to 60 degrees, causing right buttocks pain and loss of sensation in the lateral aspect of the right foot.

Chemonucleolysis with collagenase was performed at the fifth lumbar disc level. Ten days after injection, the patient developed a sciatic scoliosis (list) of 30 degrees to the left, which persisted despite some improvement in right straight leg raising to 50 degrees, causing pain referral to the right buttocks. The patient had persistent difficulty walking because of fatigue, back pain, and the list. A disc excision was performed; findings included no disc in the interspace between the vertebrae but two sequestrated fragments of disc in the spinal canal, one in the axilla of the S-1 nerve root and the other lateral to the S-1 nerve root ganglia. Histologic examination of these fragments and some residual small pieces of nucleus pulposus removed from the interspace revealed nothing unusual when compared to discs from patients who had not undergone previous collagenase injection. Intraoperative somatosensory-evoked potentials showed a decrease in latency and improvement in waveform after removal of the fragments. There was no evidence of deleterious effect of the enzyme on the tissues in the epidural space. The night following surgery, the patient walked unassisted without a list and with no leg pain. He was discharged on the third postoperative day and returned to work after 6 weeks, without a list. Plate 9 is an artist's interpretation of the reason for failure of enzyme to work in this patient. The enzyme did not reach the sequestrated fragments. The list that appeared after injection is thought to be secondary to disc space narrowing and a nonspecific proprioceptive neuromuscular reflex.

According to Bromley,[3] a sequestrated fragment of disc in the spinal canal occurs in 13% of patients operated on for disc displacement. We would agree with Bromley's estimate, particularly in a highly selected group of patients subjected to treatment on the basis of hard organic findings. In a poorly selected group of patients, a lower percentage of free disc fragments would be found. With more sophisticated computer-assisted tomography and high-resolution cuts, along with three-dimensional reconstruction, preoperative diagnosis of a sequestrated disc fragment will probably become more commonplace. We now use the following criteria to predict the presence of a sequestrated fragment of disc: a mixed root lesion, i.e., both L-5 and S-1 nerve root deficit, and an extradural defect bridging more than 3 cm on the CT scan. When the patient has these signs, we advise surgery instead of chemonucleolysis.

A more common reason for enzyme not reaching the offending disc material is that, on intradiscal injection, the fluid follows the path of least resistance, which in some instances may not be into the disc protrusion. We think that this is the most common reason for failure following chemonucleolysis. The patient described in Case 2 illustrates just such a situation (Plates 10 and 11).

CASE 2.—Thirty-three-year-old waitress with a 3-month history of low back and left leg pain of insidious onset had been treated with 1 month of bedrest at home before entering the University of Miami Hospital and Clinics in January 1982. She was in good general health. Her only complaint was disabling left leg pain.

On physical examination, in addition to a sciatic scoliosis of 20 degrees to the right, she could flex forward only 20 degrees while standing. She had a positive crossed straight leg raising of 60 degrees on the right, causing left posterior thigh pain; straight leg raising on the left at 10 degrees caused severe left leg pain. The left Achilles tendon reflex was absent.

A metrizamide myelogram showed a large extradural defect at the fifth lumbar interspace on the left consistent with an extruded disc.

On February 4, 1982 chemonucleolysis with collagenase at the fifth lumbar interspace caused partial relief of pain, list, and contralateral straight leg raising by the evening after injection. At 8-week follow-up, the patient had a persistent list of 20 degrees to the right, although straight leg raising had improved to 80 degrees on the left and to 110 degrees on the right. Forward flexion was improved to 45 degrees, but the left Achilles tendon reflex was still absent.

Since she could not return to work because of muscle spasms, fatigue, and severe sciatic scoliosis, the patient underwent a lumbar disc excision at the L-5 level on April 14, 1982. A large herniated nucleus pulposus under a pseudocapsule formed by the last few layers of the annulus fibrosus, posterior longitudinal ligament, and periosteum of the adjacent vertebra was found at surgery. When the pseudocapsule was incised, the nucleus pulposus extruded under pressure. Very little soft and friable nucleus pulposus was encountered in the disc space. Histologic examination showed fibrocartilage and was not unusual. There was no evidence of deleterious effect of collagenase on adjacent tissues. The reason for failure in this case was the failure of the enzyme to reach the herniated nucleus pulposus matrix. The patient's sciatic list gradually improved over 6 weeks following surgery, and she returned to two jobs at that time. She has had an excellent result to date.

If, on injecting dye under fluoroscopy, the dye flows into the vertebral bodies, vascular channels, or an anterior lateral defect without properly filling the area corresponding to the disc protrusion seen by myelography and/or CAT scan, one may anticipate this type of failure.[4]

WRONG LEVEL

We have seen the situation where a disc protrusion that we thought clinically significant was injected at one level and the patient failed to respond. Subsequently, at surgery, disc displacement was found at the adjacent level. We do not advocate routine multiple disc injections. However, when there is a suspected clinically significant disc displacement at more than one level, all levels suspected should be injected with dye to confirm the necessity for subsequent enzyme injection.

FAILURE OF THE ENZYME TO WORK

Not Enough Enzyme

In the original double-blind study, we were of the opinion that 1 ml containing 4 mg of chymopapain was not enough to effectively decompress the herniated disc. We think it is critical to inject a minimum of 1 cc containing 4 mg of the enzyme.[5]

The minimum effective intradiscal dosage of collagenase has not been determined. However, an effective dosage range between 500 and 600 units in a volume of 1–2 cc has effectively produced disc narrowing and at least a 75% chance of a satisfactory clinical outcome.[6]

Inactive Enzyme

Enzymes can be inactivated in transport or during storage, and specific instructions for their storage, reconstitution, and dilution should be followed precisely. For example, it is important to dilute chymopapain with sterile water without preservatives.[7] Also, alcohol should not be used to disinfect the vial prior to withdrawing the enzyme. The interaction of various contrast dyes with chymopapain has been studied by Naylor et al.[8] We also studied the interaction of iothalamate with Discase with respect to its action on human nucleus pulposus in vitro. We had results similar to Naylor's: there was no inhibition of chymopapain by iothalamate[9] (see Chap. 8).

We have also performed studies (see Chap. 8) on the interaction of various substances with collagenase. We found no evidence of inhibition of the action of collagenase by 60% iothalamate. Disc narrowing and clinically satisfactory outcome in patients are independent of whether a discogram precedes the use of collagenase.

Lateral Recess Stenosis

Symptoms from disc narrowing following chemonucleolysis resulting in foramenal or lateral recess stenosis rarely occur. More commonly, the patient suffered from some component of nerve impingement resulting from these conditions before injection. We have found this to be true in most instances. Failure to obtain relief is not due to aggravation of a pre-existing condition, but to misdiagnosis and poor patient selection. It is imperative that the surgeon understand the clinical manifestations of the various pathophysiologic consequences of disc degeneration on the motion segment unit, in order to avoid failures caused by misdiagnosis of the true cause of nerve root compression.[10]

Mechanical Insufficiency

Mechanical insufficiency of the motion segment unit rarely develops as the result of chemonucleolysis. We have, however, seen two instances in which patients developed degenerative spondylolisthesis following chemonucleolysis. In the first case, a young woman was injected at the third lumbar interspace with an excellent result for 1 year, after which she was reinjured in an accident. She developed a recurrent herniated disc and subsequently underwent a laminectomy and disc excision at the same level as the chemonucleolysis. One year after surgery she sustained yet another traumatic injury to her lower back and subsequently developed mechanical back pain[11] and a degenerative spondylolisthesis at the same level as previous chemonucleolysis and surgery.

Another patient had had previous successful laminectomy and disc excision at L4-5 and subsequently developed symptoms of a recurrent herniated disc. Chemonucleolysis at the same level relieved the leg pain; however, the patient developed degenerative spondylolisthesis and persistent mechanical back pain.

These are highly unusual cases, and the development of mechanical insufficiency was probably independent of the chemonucleolysis.

We are seeing dramatic disc space narrowing as the result of collagenase injection. It remains to be determined whether collagenase will predispose patients to mechanical insufficiency of the motion segment unit. Conversely, it is possible that collagenase injection may prove to be an efficient method of stabilizing the intervertebral joint by stimulating narrowing and subsequent new collagen formation.

Acute Facet Symptoms

Following chemonucleolysis, an occasional patient has developed transient leg pain on the side opposite the original sciatica. None of these patients have developed signs of nerve root tension or compression. All of them have had a nonspecific sclerotogenous referral of pain, which has resolved over a period of weeks. Contralateral leg pain in the absence of nerve root compromise has not been a cause for permanent failure of chemonucleolysis, in our experience. The referred leg pain probably occurs because of narrowing of the interspace, with subsequent subluxation of the facet joint processes, cartilaginous erosion, and reactive synovitis in the synovial facet joint capsule. Time, a lumbar support, and anti-inflammatory medication with graduated exercise will help to alleviate leg pain that results from acute disc space narrowing. Referral pain of this nature has resolved within 3 months of injection in every patient.

WHEN TO OPERATE

In the absence of absolute indications, how long does one wait before performing surgery following chemonucleolysis? If after 6 weeks, the patient has had no improvement of spinal flexion, straight leg raising or femoral stretching, neurologic deficit, pain relief, or increased activity, then surgery is indicated.

There are patients who, despite persistent pain, have improvement in their physical findings at 6 weeks. We have encouraged them to wait even longer and have subsequently seen them go on to a good or excellent symptomatic result with an additional 6 weeks of observation. Occasionally at 6 weeks' follow-up, a patient has slight symptomatic improvement as the result of inactivity and rest, but no improvement in physical findings. When this occurs, we recommend surgery (see Case 2).

Increasing Neurologic Deficit

We have not seen a patient who has required immediate surgical decompression after chemonucleolysis because of rapid deterioration of neurologic function. It is surprising that the literature and numerous personal communications concerning more than 20,000 patients treated with chymopapain and 200 treated with collagenase have failed to document any such cases. However, caution should be exercised when considering chemonucleolysis for patients complaining of urinary hesitancy or urgency or urinary retention with back pain—particularly when the myelogram and/or CAT scan reveals a central disc displacement of a significant degree. The use of common sense in patient selection and avoidance of patients with disabling neurologic deficit (or the potential for such), is imperative to prevent sudden massive neurologic deterioration following an intradiscal injection.

In rare instances, an intradiscal injection could potentiate a disc extrusion or protrusion thus leading to rapid increase in neurologic deficit. Should this occur, surgery is indicated immediately.

We had one patient who, upon injection, had increased sciatica with weakness in the extensor hallucis longus. The patient subsequently had relief of sciatica, a return of the Achilles tendon reflex, and loss of hypesthesia on the lateral aspect of the foot, but persistent weakness of the big-toe extensor. We did not consider this patient as a failure of treatment, although a new neurologic deficit occurred. The patient had relief of neural compression of the first sacral nerve root as the result of intradiscal enzyme injection but developed persistent fifth motor nerve root deficit. This sequence may have been caused by the intradiscal injection mechanically displacing an extruded disc fragment off the first sacral nerve root and onto the fifth lumbar nerve root. This is an interesting case because, despite an excellent clinical result, the patient experienced a slight deterioration of motor nerve root function.

OUR FAILURES WITH CHYMOPAPAIN

Of 49 patients that we have managed with injection of chymopapain, we have operated on eight (16%). The median interval between enzyme injection to surgery was 7 weeks. Two patients had a lateral recess stenosis as the major cause of persistent radiculopathy. They were treated before sophisticated CAT scan and water-soluble myelography techniques were available. In three patients, chymopapain did not dissolve the disc for the various reasons mentioned above. Two patients had psychogenic regional pain disturbance, which in retrospect was misdiagnosed and should have been treated before choosing chemonucleolysis in the first place. The patients subsequently underwent surgery, and the full-blown psychogenic regional pain disturbance then became apparent. Failure to recognize severe pain-producing or pain-enhancing behavior is becoming a less frequent problem with our better understanding of the implications[12] of, and methods for, diagnosing[13] such disturbances.

OUR FAILURES WITH COLLAGENASE

Of 23 patients in our center who have had collagenase injections, three have undergone surgery. One patient had a sequestrated disc; and a second had a large disc protrusion that the enzyme had obviously not reached. In both these cases, the disc had narrowed after injection, and there was no appreciable nucleus pulposus left between the vertebrae. The third patient had no improvement in restricted straight leg raising, and contralateral straight leg raising continued to produce leg pain in the symptomatic side 3 months after enzyme injection into the fourth lumbar disc above a transitional vertebra. At surgery, a very hard annulus protrusion was found in one axilla of the fifth lumbar nerve root. The disc space itself had very little residual nucleus pulposus. There was no evidence in any of these patients of a deleterious effect of collagenase on surrounding tissues.

We have had no case of failure of collagenase due to misdiagnosis of a tumor, infection, facet osteoarthritis, mechanical insufficiency, or spinal stenosis.

COMPLICATIONS

Complications from chemonucleolysis can be limited by excellent patient selection, preinjection rehabilitation, and careful attention to technique as previously outlined in Chapter 6. Despite the best patient selection and technique, there will be a small percentage of unavoidable complications. Sensitivity reactions, although usually transient and not leading to permanent morbidity, are the most common of the unavoidable complications and potentially the most serious. A detailed discussion of the mechanism, diagnosis, and management of sensitivity reactions is in order.

SENSITIVITY REACTIONS WITH CHYMOPAPAIN

There were 201 sensitivity reactions in the first 13,700 patients treated with chymopapain (1.5%) of which 53 were mild, 52 moderate, and 25 severe immediate systemic reactions.[14]

We are concerned with the management of immediate systemic allergic reactions, 25 of which were severe, an incidence of 0.2%. Two of these patients died.

The most recent statistics (October 1982) available are based upon 40,000 patients injected with chymopapain. There have been a total of four fatalities from anaphylaxis caused by chymopapain, an incidence of 0.01%.

When anaphylactic reactions are severe and common to a drug, discontinuing its use may be justified.[15] The efficacy of the drug must be determined in relation to the frequency of unfavorable reactions. In the case of chymopapain, a 1% reaction rate is relatively high. It is estimated that penicillin injection is responsible for 0.002%[16] fatality rate, whereas urographic contrast medium has a 0.001% fatality rate.[17] Compare these figures with the 0.01% fatality rate for chymopapain, and it appears that chymopapain is a riskier drug than x-ray contrast dye and penicillin. No matter what the figures show, a death from anaphylaxis in a non-life-threatening disease such as disc displacement is a catastrophy to all involved.

We are of the opinion that, with proper precautions (patient preparation, prophylaxis, early recognition and prompt management of reactions), chymopapain is safer than the present fatality statistics indicate. The following discussion explores anaphylaxis in depth to substantiate this statement.

CHYMOPAPAIN ANAPHYLAXIS: TWO FATAL CASES

DiMaio[18] reported the case histories of two patients, both of whom were treated under general anesthesia without an endotracheal tube. The first patient, a 45-year-old female, was given general anesthesia and was premedicated with 100 mg of Solu-Cortef and 25 mg of Benadryl intramuscularly. A discogram was done with Renografin; after 10 minutes, 1 ml of chymopapain was injected. *Four minutes* later, the patient developed "gooseflesh" (cutis anserina) and hypotension. The blood pressure was unobtainable. The patient was given 100 mg of Solu-Cortef and 25 mg of Benadryl intravenously. (Epinephrine and large volumes of IV fluids should be administered here.) One hour and 35 minutes later, she was dead.

In the second case, DiMaio reports a 25-year-old female was injected with chymopapain under Penthrane general anesthesia with an endotracheal tube in place. Preanesthesia medication included 50 mg of Solu-Cortef and 25 mg of Benadryl intramuscularly. The patient had a two-level discogram with Renografin; 15 minutes later 1 ml of chymopapain was injected into the L-5 disc. *Immediately* following the injection, the anesthesiologist noted erythema characterized by a warm sensation of the skin and gooseflesh. The blood pressure then became unobtainable. The patient was treated with Regitine, a vasopressor. (Epinephrine is used to block mediators of anaphylaxis, not to support blood pressure.) Despite the usual supportive measures, the patient continued to have unobtainable blood pressure for 12 hours. Twenty-four hours after the reaction, with a blood pressure of 60/20, the patient developed acute abdominal signs and symptoms and was taken to the operating room for an exploratory laparotomy. She was found to have an infarction of the small bowel and ascending colon. The patient died on the operating table.

Neither of these two patients received the specific antidote for anaphylactic reactions—epinephrine early in the reaction and massive infusion of intravenous fluids to support the blood pressure.

POSTMORTEM FINDINGS IN FATAL ANAPHYLAXIS

Edema of the airway in man is a feature of anaphylaxis unique to our species. Typical of autopsy findings on 43 patients reported by Delage and Irey[19] was distention of the lungs with laryngeal edema and pulmonary emphysema. The majority of the patients were young people treated with penicillin. These patients usually manifest respiratory distress followed by circulatory collapse. Occasionally, seizures, cyanosis, and gastrointestinal symptoms are the first signs of fatal anaphylaxis. The interval between injection and onset of the reaction was less than 20 minutes in 86% (37 out of 43) of cases where anaphylaxis resulted in death. The time from onset to death was 30 minutes in 14 of the 43 cases.

CASE REPORTS OF
NONFATAL ANAPHYLAXIS TO CHYMOPAPAIN

Anaphylaxis Under Anesthesia

An anaphylactic reaction to chymopapain during anesthesia was reported by Rajagopalan et al.[20] A 48-year-old woman under general endotracheal anesthesia, including thiopental, nitrous oxide, and oxygen, was given an antihistamine (chlorpheniramine, 10 mg) and 100 mg of hydrocortisone intravenously after induction of anesthesia. Discography was performed, and 10 minutes later 10,000 units of chymopapain was injected intradiscally. Anesthesia was reversed. The patient was extubated and *15 minutes* after injection, a routine check of blood pressure showed an unobtainable pressure. One hundred percent oxygen was administered by mask and 800 ml of intravenous fluid was administered rapidly, along with methoxamine 4 + 4 g. One milliliter of 1:10,000 epinephrine solution was given intravenously after the electrocardiogram showed a normal pattern with a heart rate of 80 beats per minute. Im-

mediately after receiving epinephrine, the patient had frequent premature ventricular contractions. She developed facial and periorbital
edema and mild generalized bronchospasms. Fifteen minutes after the
onset of the reaction, her systolic blood pressure was 90 mm Hg; and,
although she was stuporous for several hours, she recovered completely
within 10 hours.

In this patient, premedications were Benadryl and hydrocortisone, the
hypotension was treated with intravenous fluids, and the reaction was
managed with 1 ml of epinephrine. She had received gallamine in pref-
erence to curare as a muscle relaxant, since the former releases less
histamine than the latter. The anesthesiologist avoided using halothane
for fear of potentiating a cardiac arrhythmia, should epinephrine be
needed for anaphylactoid reaction. Rajagopalan suggested that isoproterenol (Isuprel) may be a safer β-adrenergic agonist than epinephrine,
which causes cardiac arrhythmias. However, Isuprel does potentiate hypotension. All the preventive measures in this case may have helped
avoid a tragic outcome.

Other Case Reports With General Anesthesia

Clark Watts et al.[21] reported on four patients who had immediate systemic sensitivity reactions typical of anaphylaxis after chymopapain injections during general anesthesia. All four had been induced with sodium thiopental, paralyzed with succinylcholine, and intubated. General anesthesia was maintained with halothane and oxygen. Discograms
were performed in one to three levels with Renografin.

The first patient, a 66-year-old man, developed hypotension within
minutes after injection of 4 mg of chymopapain. He had a mild systemic
reaction with a blood pressure of 70/50, which responded immediately to
25 mg of intravenous ephedrine. Over the next 2 hours, additional do-
sages of ephedrine were given to maintain normal blood pressure. The
patient had received 100 mg of hydrocortisone and 50 mg of diphenhydramine intramuscularly before injection. He was receiving hydrocortisone at the time of the chymopapain injection. He had an uneventful
recovery within 2 hours.

The second patient, a 60-year-old woman, had a cutaneous, petechiae-
like eruption within minutes after 4 mg of chymopapain was injected.
This would be classified as a mild systemic allergic reaction. She was
treated with intravenous hydrocortisone with no problem.

The third case is that of a 25-year-old woman who had hypotension
and generalized urticaria *within minutes* after injection of 4 mg of chymopapain into the L-4 disc and 4 mg into the L-5 disc. She developed
hypotension and pulmonary wheezes and was treated with hydrocortisone and epinephrine intravenously over the next few hours. She had
not received preinjection steroids. After 4 hours, her condition stabilized.

The fourth patient, a 32-year-old woman, had tachycardia and hypotension within *2 minutes* after injection of 4 mg of chymopapain. This was immediately treated with 25 mg of ephedrine intravenously. Within 3 minutes, her blood pressure was unobtainable; 0.3 milliliters of a 1:1,000 solution of epinephrine was given intravenously. Within 3 minutes, a previously unpalpable femoral pulse and carotid pulse were discernible. Intravenous fluids were administered rapidly because no brachial pulse could be recorded. Over the next 2 hours, 4 L of balanced salt solution was given. The patient was under Innovar anesthesia with nitrous oxide inhalant. Immediately after the hypotensive episode, the patient was placed on pure oxygen but remained comatose for 45 minutes. It was an hour before urinary output resumed. Two hours later, blood pressure had returned to 100/70 mm Hg. Twelve hours after injection of chymopapain, she became asymptomatic. She had received hydrocortisone and diphenhydramine as preoperative medications intramuscularly.

A Case Report Without General Anesthesia

I reported a case of a 32-year-old male who, after discography with Conray-60 at two levels was injected with chymopapain at both levels. In *one minute,* he developed severe back and bilateral leg pain; tingling in the arms, hands, feet, and perioral region; followed rapidly by pruritis and urticaria. The patient rapidly developed perioral pallor, dyspnea, and stridor. One-half milliliter of a 1:10,000 epinephrine solution was administered intravenously, along with several liters of Ringer's lactate. Within 10 minutes the patient had recovered, but he experienced headaches for several hours following the procedure. This patient had been premedicated one-half hour before the procedure with 50 mg of Benadryl and 100 mg of hydrocortisone intramuscularly and injected under local anesthesia with intravenous fluids running. In this case, a small dose of epinephrine, administered within 60 seconds of onset of anaphylaxis, was sufficient to abort the attack. The reaction was rapidly recognized under local anesthesia.

WHAT IS ANAPHYLAXIS?

Anaphylaxis in man is a systemic symptom complex resulting from antigen-antibody interaction.[22] The patient must have been exposed to the antigen at some time in the past so that IgE antibody is attached to the mast cells in the target organs (lung, gastrointestinal tract, and skin). With reinjection of antigen at various periods following sensitization, an antigen-antibody complex occurs on the surface of the mast cells, causing a massive release of the pharmacologic mediators: histamine, slow-reacting substance of anaphylaxis (SRS-A), serotonin, and bradykinin. These mediators then act on the target organs.

Mediators

Histamine, thought to be the major mediator of anaphylaxis in man, causes bronchial constriction and increases capillary permeability. Slow-reacting substance of anaphylaxis (SRS-A) causes bronchial smooth muscle contraction in humans.[22] It is also responsible for increased vascular permeability. Bradykinin causes vasodilatation, compounds the effects of histamine, increases capillary permeability, and is thought to be the primary substance in man responsible for the severe hypotension noted.

The mediators may cause a greatly variable response in different patients. The major targets in humans are smooth muscles, which, on contraction, may cause severe bronchiolar constriction resulting in asphyxia, increased peripheral arterial resistance secondary to vasoconstriction, nausea and vomiting secondary to smooth muscle contraction in the bowel, and "gooseflesh" (cutis anserina) from contraction of the pilar erectae muscles in the skin.

The severe fall in arterial blood pressure is secondary to a decline in cardiac output and a loss of fluid from the intravascular space due to increased capillary permeability. Shock is due to reduced plasma volume, hemoconcentration, decreased cardiac output, reduced peripheral blood flow, and increased arterial constriction. It is very important to remember that hypotension is due to intravascular fluid loss due to increased capillary permeability.

Acute vascular collapse from anaphylaxis is secondary to cardiac arrhythmias, acute myocardial infarction, and vasomotor collapse. Direct cardiac anaphylaxis is secondary to the direct action of the chemical mediators on the myocardium and may be compounded by epinephrine, halothane, and pre-existing heart disease.

Abnormal electrocardiograms have been noted within 24 hours of the onset of systemic anaphylaxis in six of 14 patients.[23] None had pre-existing heart disease. ECG changes may be the result of the direct effect of mediators on the myocardium and/or the compounding effects of epinephrine and anesthetic agents. Pre-existing occult heart disease with superimposed stress may also be implicated when abnormal ECGs occur.

Knowledge of the manifestations, potential immediate disastrous effects, and pathophysiology of anaphylaxis will help us make decisions concerning prophylaxis and management of this complication.

Prevention of Anaphylaxis

There are no reliable tests to predict whether a patient will experience an immediate systemic sensitivity reaction. Some reactions can be prevented by carefully noting a history of allergy to papaya, meat tenderizer containing papain, or previous injection with chymopapain. Previous allergic reaction to burn ointments containing collagenase or previous collagenase injection should also be sought in the history if this enzyme is to be given. Avoid injecting these patients.

Prophylaxis

In Wiltse's series of 1,200 patients,[24] the first 600 were not pretreated with antihistamines and steroids. There were seven serious allergic reactions. The second 600 patients were pretreated with antihistamine and steroids; and there were two serious systemic allergic reactions, neither of which seemed as severe as the previous seven. It remains to be determined whether the use of antihistamines and steroids as a prophylactic measure decreases the incidence and severity of anaphylactic reactions. However, there is some circumstantial evidence from several series in the literature concerning the reactions to contrast media in patients who had prior adverse reactions.

Kelly et al.[25] reported on 101 patients who had prior anaphylactoid reactions to contrast media and who were pretreated with prednisone and diphenhydramine 1 hour before a repeat diagnostic study with a contrast media. Five of the 101 patients (5%) developed a systemic sensitivity reaction, characterized by mild urticaria and pruritis. There were no life-threatening reactions in this high-risk group of patients. In an earlier study of 115 patients, there was a 30% recurrence of serious anaphylactic reactions in patients who had had previous reactions to contrast media.[26] The data seem to suggest that antihistamines and hydrocortisone effectively reduce the risk of an anaphylactic reaction in the patient who has been presensitized with an antigen. The fact that Kelly et al. have found no significant life-threatening anaphylactic reactions in those patients, despite their previous systemic sensitivity reactions, is highly significant. There is evidence that pretreatment steroids and antihistamines in Wiltse's series protected the patients against anaphylaxis. However, surgeons should not be lulled into complacency when pretreatment has been given. Such precautions may give the patient an advantage, but early recognition of anaphylaxis, epinephrine, and intravenous fluids are still essential.

H_1 AND H_2 ANTAGONIST FOR ANAPHYLAXIS

During initial clinical trials of Chymodiactin (chymopapain), two patients suffered fatal anaphylactic reactions. Following this, the investigators extensively reviewed current literature on the cardiovascular effects of systemic allergic reaction.

One of the mediators of anaphylaxis, histamine, acts on two receptors, H_1 and H_2, both of which appear in the heart and peripheral vasculature. Theoretically, the administration of an antagonist to both receptors may afford some protection against the cardiovascular effects of histamine release after anaphylactic reactions. Prospective double-blind studies have shown that administration of H_1 (diphenhydramine) and H_2 (cimetidine) protected patients from the hemodynamic effect of histamine release after intravenous administration of morphine.[27]

The use of cimetidine, 300 mg by mouth every 6 hours for 24 hours, and diphenhydramine (Benadryl), 50 mg by mouth every 6 hours for 24 hours, before injection of chymopapain is now advocated.[28] We appreciate the theoretical basis for this suggestion but caution physicians against depending on any unproved method for preventing the serious consequences of an anaphylactic reaction. One must still be prepared to make an immediate diagnosis and administer adrenaline and large amounts of fluid, should an anaphylactic reaction occur. Hopefully, pretreatment with cimetidine and diphenhydramine will be effective protection against the disastrous hemodynamic effects of a severe systemic allergic reaction.

Early Recognition

John McCulloch[29] who treated 5,000 patients by injection with Discase, reported 15 patients with acute severe anaphylactic reactions. He stated that the onset is varied: some patients have a precipitous fall in blood pressure followed by cutaneous manifestations; others have tingling, paresthesia, flush, wheezing, and then falling blood pressure. All his patients were injected under local anesthesia, with an anesthesiologist in attendance. McCulloch's experience in successful management of anaphylaxis is probably the most extensive in the world. He emphasizes the importance of early recognition and the immediate administration of epinephrine and intravenous fluids. None of his patients had permanent sequelae of immediate systemic sensitivity reactions to chymopapain.

Choice of Anesthesia

We advocate the use of local anesthesia so that we can recognize any reaction early and avoid the compounding effects of anesthesia on the reaction itself and on epinephrine administration.

An anesthesiologist should attend every patient, even when local anesthesia is used. A blood pressure cuff should be in place, IV fluid running, and a cardiac monitor in place. The anesthesiologist should be fully aware of the risks of anaphylaxis and its management. The entire procedure should be a team effort of both surgeon and anesthesiologist.

Prior discussion of risks and coordinated acute care for any anaphylactic reaction may mean the difference between life and death.

The Clinical Picture

Usually, symptoms begin within the first 2 minutes after antigen injection. Sudden and extreme hypotension is noted in potentially fatal reactions. In these instances, treatment must begin within seconds.

One word of caution: if the patient is improving after initial therapy with epinephrine and intravenous fluids, do not let your guard down. Epinephrine is a short-acting drug. Keep an eye on the patient for at least 24 hours. The duration of the reaction is variable from patient to patient and may last up to 24 hours, despite intensive immediate therapy. Wheezing, hypotension, and other symptoms may last for days. The intensity of the reaction, the time of onset following therapy, and the duration of symptoms vary greatly from patient to patient.

Another word of caution: norephinephrine (ephedrine) enhances release of the mediators and may be contraindicated in the treatment of anaphylaxis. Since isoproterenol inhibits mediator release and may serve as a potent bronchodilator, it may be a good alternative to epinephrine. Other vasopressors, such as Regitine, etc., are contraindicated. The absolute antidote for anaphylaxis is the administration of epinephrine before irreversible end-organ response to the mediators. This is critical, since late administration will compound the cardiovascular toxicity already present from the direct effect of mediators and from the secondary effects of anoxia due to decreased cardiac output and massive vasodilatation.

LATE MANIFESTATIONS OF SYSTEMIC SENSITIVITY

It is important to realize that anaphylaxis may occur up to 2 hours after exposure to the antigen, particularly with intradiscal enzyme injection. Since the disc is avascular, it may take several hours for chymopapain to be released into the bloodstream; hence the possibility of delayed anaphylaxis. It is imperative to monitor these patients for 30 minutes after injection and in the recovery room for an additional hour. After 2 hours, the risk of severe systemic allergic reaction is remote. The half-life of breakdown products of chymopapain is approximately one week. This fact may account for delayed sensitivity reactions that have manifested as benign cutaneous reactions 10 days to 3 weeks after injection. Such reactions are easily managed by a few days' treatment with antihistamines. No patient has experienced permanent sequelae from these reactions. It is important, however, to warn patients to avoid papaya or meat tenderizers containing papaya enzymes in the future.

COMPLICATIONS OTHER THAN ALLERGY

Neural Injury

Neural injury can be avoided by performing the procedure under local anesthesia and redirecting the needle when the patient complains of acute radicular pain. The nerve root or ganglia injured by needle penetrations is usually the one above the root or ganglia being injured by disc displacement (Plate 7). Note the needle entering the posterior lateral corner of the L5-S1 disc. The proximity of the L-5 root ganglia and nerve root can be seen. If the patient is suffering from S-1 radiculopathy secondary to lumbosacral disc displacement, the L-5 root is in jeopardy from intradiscal injection.

If causalgia, increased nerve root pain, and/or neurologic deficit occur from needle puncture, the only therapy is time and symptomatic treatment. The patient should be reassured that, in most instances, symptoms and signs will resolve with time.

Cardiovascular Complications

Avoidance of high-risk patients and appropriate preinjection prophylaxis will help to decrease the incidence of these complications. A certain small incidence of cardiovascular complications, such as thromboembolic phenomena, cerebral vascular accidents, and myocardial infarctions will occur during the course of treatment in any group of patients under stress. There are fewer of these complications with chemonucleolysis versus surgery; and if they do occur, they are more easily managed after chemonucleolysis than after surgery.

CASE 3.—A 52-year-old male physician developed acute low back pain and left leg pain in March 1975. He had suffered low back strain in 1952 with intermittent mild recurrences since. Left-sided sciatica had recurred 3 weeks before his admission to the University of Miami Hospital and Clinics on March 28, 1975. The patient had been in bed, on narcotics, 1 day prior to admission. He had been treated for hypertensive cardiovascular disease in the past. Findings on admission included a positive straight leg raising 40 degrees left, with pain referral to the buttocks. Cross straight leg raising 40 degrees right caused left leg pain to the ankle. There was no left Achilles tendon reflex, no sensation in the lateral aspect of the left foot, and ipsilateral weakness of the anterior tibial muscle. A myelogram demonstrated a lateral extradural defect at the fifth lumbar interspace on the left, consistent with disc displacement.

On April 2, 1975, the patient was premedicated with atropine 0.4 mg, hydrocortisone, and Benadryl. Before discography, a left bundle branch block (LBBB) was noted on the cardiac monitor. The procedure was cancelled. The patient was observed at bedrest for the next 12 days. Enzyme studies (CPK, SGPT, and LDH) were normal. ECG showed persistent LBBB.

On April 14, 1975 discography confirmed the diagnosis of a fifth lumbar disc herniation. Discase injection was followed within minutes by subjective relief of paresthesia in the left foot. Straight leg raising and crossed straight leg raising were negative at 90 degrees. The patient required no further narcotics. He noted mild right anterior chest pain, which was attributed to his position on the x-ray table before discography. The following morning, the chest pain persisted and was pleuritic in nature. Chest x-ray revealed a right middle lobe infiltrate. Arterial blood gas (55 mg%) readings confirmed the diagnosis of pulmonary embolism. A lung scan was positive. The patient was treated with nasal oxygen, anticoagulants, and rest and was discharged April 26, 1975, improved.

Five weeks after injection, patient returned to work, had negative straight leg raising but persistently absent Achilles tendon reflex and decreased sensation in the lateral aspect of the left foot. There were no motor deficits. On September 3, 1975 the patient remained asymptomatic, at work, but had occasional paresthesia in the left foot. He was of the opinion that the innocuous nature of the chemonucleolysis treatment, as compared to surgery, saved his life. We agreed with an internist consultant that the pulmonary embolism occurred before injection, but first became symptomatic on the day of injection.

We do not advocate chemonucleolysis in lieu of surgery for disc displacement in high-risk patients with medical problems. The stress of anaphylaxis, had it occurred in this patient, could have been lethal. We would never have injected this patient had we suspected pulmonary embolism. We would now begin detoxification from pain medication and ambulation before undertaking elective intradiscal therapy in a patient subjected to prolonged bedrest due to medical problems.

Neural Toxicity

Intrathecal Injection of Enzyme

We try to avoid intrathecal injection of enzyme by performing a discogram prior to enzyme injection. Although a case of intrathecal enzyme injection as the result of a pre-existing intrathecal disc herniation has not been reported, it could occur; and one should pay attention to the contrast dye flow pattern before enzyme injection. Enzyme should be injected via the lateral approach only, never by the posterolateral route, to avoid nerve root penetration and intrathecal injection (Plate 12).

If the patient complains of severe headache, back pain, and leg pain in conjunction with signs of increased intracranial pressure, an emergency spinal tap and repeated taps are in order to decrease the intrathecal cerebral spinal fluid pressure. Elevation of cerebral spinal fluid pressure occurs secondary to hemorrhage.

Discitis and Disc Space Infection

Most patients have some acute narrowing of the intervertebral disc in the postinjection period with either chymopapain or collagenase. After an initial period ranging from 2 to 4 weeks of increased back pain, the patient should improve progressively between 4 and 7 weeks after injection. Increased pain accompanied by sleep disturbances and muscle spasm during this period should alert the surgeon to a possible disc space infection. Close adherence to proper injection technique, should make this complication extremely rare. Early confirmation of the diagnosis can be made by a positive bone scan. Later in the course of the disease, after 2–3 weeks of increasing symptoms, the patient's x-rays may show erosion of the bony end plates of the vertebral bodies adjacent to the disc space in question. There may be an elevated sedimentation rate and white blood cell count, with a shift of the differential count to the left. A closed Craig needle biopsy, culture, and sensitivity and histologic confirmation of the diagnosis should be performed as soon as a disc space infection is suspected. Six weeks of specific intravenous antibiotic therapy, followed by 6 months of oral antibiotics, are indicated to eradicate this type of infection in an avascular space.[30]

REFERENCES

1. Smith L.: Failures with chemonucleolysis. *Orthop. Clin. North Am.* 1:255, 1975.
2. McCulloch J.A.: Chemonucleolysis. *J. Bone Joint Surg.* 59:45, 1977.
3. Bromley J.: Clinical and Double Blind Studies Concerning Collagenase. Paper presented to Deidesheimes Gespräch, Deidesheim, Germany, 1982.
4. Brown M.D., Panjabi M., Lindahl S., et al.: Measurement of disc degeneration by simultaneous volume and pressure recordings during discography. Read before the International Society for the Study of the Lumbar Spine, Toronto, June 1982.
5. Report of the Committee on Chymopapain (Discase). Chicago, American Academy of Orthopaedic Surgeons, 1975.
6. Bromley J.: Intervertebral Discolysis with Collagenase. Paper presented to International Society for the Study of the Lumbar Spine, Paris, 1981.
7. Saunders E.C.: Treatment of the canine intervertebral disc syndrome with chymopapain. *J. Am. Vet. Med. Assoc.* 145:893, 1964.
8. Naylor A., Earland C., Robinson J.: The effect of diagnostic radio-opaque fluids used in discography on chymopapain activity. *Spine,* accepted for publication, 1983.
9. Brown M.D., Ramos M.: In vitro effects of chymopapain, iothalamate and EDTA on human nucleus pulposus. Dept. of Orthopedics and Rehabilitation, University of Miami School of Medicine, August 1980.

10. Grabias S.: The treatment of spinal stenosis. *J. Bone Joint Surg.* 42A:308, 1980.
11. Brown M.D.: Lumbar spine fusion, in Finneson B.E. (ed.): *Low Back Pain,* ed. 2. Philadelphia, J.B. Lippincott Co., 1979.
12. Wiltse L.L., Rocchio P.D.: Preoperative psychological tests as predictors of success of chemonucleolysis in the treatment of the low back syndrome. *J. Bone Joint Surg.* 57A:478, 1975.
13. Waddell G., McCulloch J., Kummel E., Venny R.: Nonorganic physical signs in low back pain. *Spine* 5:11, 1980.
14. Watts C.: Complications of chemonucleolysis for lumbar disc disease. *Neurosurgery* 1:2, 1977.
15. Kern R.A.: Anaphylactic drug reactions: Their diagnosis, prevention and treatment. *J.A.M.A.* 179:19, 1962.
16. Idsoe O., Guthrie T., Willcox R.R., DeWeck A.L.: Nature and extent of penicillin side-reactions with particular reference to fatalities from anaphylactic shock. *Bull. WHO* 38:159, 1968.
17. Kaplan R.: Sensitivity reaction—chymopapain vs. radiographic dye (letter). Anesthesiology 47:399, 1977.
18. DiMaio V.J.: Two anaphylactic deaths after chemonucleolysis. *J. Forensic Sci.* 21:187, 1976.
19. Delage C., Irey N.: Anaphylactic deaths: A clinicopathologic study of 43 cases. *J. Forensic Sci.* 17:525, 1972.
20. Rajagopalan R., Tindal S., MacNab I.: Anaphylactic reactions to chymopapain during general anesthesia: A case report. *Anesth. Analg.* 53:191, 1974.
21. Watts C., Williams O.B., Goldstein, G.: Sensitivity reactions to intradiscal injection of chymopapain during anesthesia. *Anesthesiology* 44:43, 1976.
22. Kelly J., Patterson R.: Anaphylaxis: Course, mechanism and treatment. *J.A.M.A.* 227:1431, 1974.
23. Hanashiro P.K., Weil M.H.: Anaphylactic shock in man. *Arch. Intern. Med.* 119:129, 1967.
24. Wiltse L.L., Widell E.H., Hansen A.Y.: Chymopapain chemonucleolysis in lumbar disc disease. *J.A.M.A.* 231:474, 1975.
25. Kelly J., Patterson R., Lieberman P., et al.: Radiographic contrast media studies in high-risk patients. *J. Allergy Clin. Immunol.* 62:181, 1978.
26. Fisher H.W., Doust V.L.: An evaluation of pretesting in the problem of serious and fatal reactions to excretory venography. *Radiology* 103:497, 1972.
27. Philbin D.M., Moss J., Akins C.W., et al.: The use of H_1 and H_2 histamine antagonists with morphine anesthesia: A double-blind study. *Anesthesiology* 55:292, 1981.
28. Schoning B., Lorenz W., Doenicke A.: Prophylaxis of anaphylactoid reactions to a polypeptidal plasma substitute by H_1 plus H_2 receptor antagonists: Synopsis of three randomized controlled trials. *Klin. Wochenschr.* 60:1048, 1982.
29. McCulloch, J.S.: Personal communication, August 1982.
30. Digby J.M., Kersley J.B.: Pyogenic non-tuberculous spinal infection *J. Bone Joint Surg.* 61B:47, 1979.

8 / A Comparison of Chymopapain and Collagenase

INTRADISCAL THERAPY is a fascinating subject, not just because of the overwhelming clinical implications, but also because we can now biochemically alter connective tissue structure for therapeutic purposes. In addition to being able to chemically decompress nerves, we have gained new insights into the mechanisms of low back pain and sciatica.

ACTION OF ENZYMES ON THE PROTEOGLYCAN-COLLAGEN COMPLEX

The matrix of the nucleus pulposus contains proteoglycans and randomly dispersed collagen fibers. Chymopapain splits the protein core of the acid-aminoglycan molecules, whereas collagenase depolymerizes native collagen (Table 8–1). There is a symbiotic relationship between acid-aminoglycan and collagen macromolecules in the tissue matrix.[1]

To study this relationship further, we have taken human nucleus pulposus removed at surgery and divided it into equal fragments. The fragments have been exposed to therapeutic concentrations of either chymopapain (Discase) or collagenase (Nucleolysin) under sterile conditions at 37 C for various time intervals. There is a gross difference in the effect of the two enzymes on the disc fragments. As soon as the disc fragments are exposed to chymopapain, the supranatant solution becomes cloudy. The chymopapain immediately begins to release proteoglycans from the disc matrix into the supranatant. On the other hand, after exposure of the disc fragment to collagenase, the supranatant remains clear for several hours. After 12 hours' exposure, fibrous tissue fragments still remain in the test tubes containing chymopapain, whereas the tubes with collagenase show almost complete dissolution of the disc fragments.

ELECTRON MICROSCOPY

Hilda Lo, of the surgical research laboratories at the University of Miami School of Medicine, has performed transmission electron microscopy on the nucleus pulposus removed at surgery from a 32-year-old man (Fig 8–1). The control specimen demonstrates the typical electron microscopic appearance of nucleus pulposus[2] containing matrix vesi-

115

TABLE 8–1. COMPARISON OF CHYMOPAPAIN AND COLLAGENASE

	CHYMOPAPAIN	COLLAGENASE
Origin	Plant	Bacterium
Source	Papaya latex	C. histolyticum
Substrate	Protein backbone of acid aminoglycan molecule	Native collagen, Types I and II
Cell toxicity	None	None
Commercial source	Travenol Laboratories (Discase) Smith Laboratories (Chymodiactin) Ortho-Tex Laboratories (Chemolase)	Advance Biofactures (Nucleolysin)
How supplied	Lyophilized – 20 C 20 mg (10,000 units) per vial	Frozen – 20 C 600 units per vial
Effective intradiscal dose	4–8 mg per disc	300–600 units per disc
Ratio of toxic intrathecal dose to therapeutic intradiscal dose	2.0	3.0
Other uses	Clarify beer Tenderize meat In toothpaste and powder In chewing gum	Burn debridement Tissue culture preparation Tissue transplantation
Chance of prior sensitization	Approx. 1% of population	Unknown
Sensitivity	1% of 40,000 patients	0
Efficacy	80% satisfactory relief	80% satisfactory relief
Current status (1982)	Phase IV	Phase III
FDA approval	Chymodiactin to Phase IV (Nov. 1982)	Nucleolysin to Phase III (Dec. 1981)

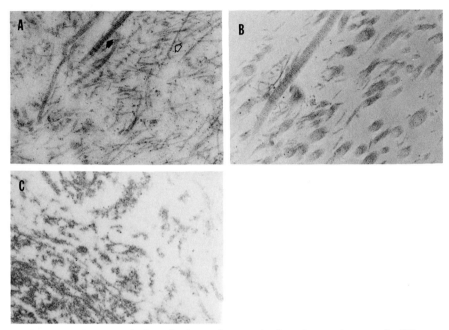

Fig 8–1.—A, transmission electron micrograph of nucleus pulposus of a 32-year-old man. Matrix of cartilage shows collagen 1 *(black arrow),* collagen 2 *(open arrow),* and small osmophilic matrix granules. × 60,000. **B,** chymopapain-treated nucleus pulposus. Note the collagens and matrix granules remained in the matrix. × 60,000. **C,** collagenase-treated nucleus pulposus. Note the amorphous structure and remaining matrix granules. No collagen or matrix vesicles were observed. × 60,000. (Courtesy of Hilda K. Lo, Surgical Research Laboratories, University of Miami School of Medicine.)

cles, randomly dispersed Type 1 and Type 2 collagen fibers, and protein polysaccharide molecules intimately associated with the collagen fibers. After exposure of another piece of the same disc sample to chymopapain, for 12 hours at 37 C under sterile conditions, one can see randomly dispersed Type 1 and Type 2 collagen fibers and a depletion of matrix vesicles. There are no discernible protein polysaccharides remaining. After exposure of a third fragment of the same sample of nucleus pulposus to collagenase at 37 C for 12 hours, an amorphous material remains. There are a few remaining matrix granules, but no collagen fibers or matrix vesicles can be seen. To obtain the sample after exposure to collagenase, the mixture had to be centrifuged, and the sediment at the bottom of the tube collected and prepared for examination by electron microscopy.

We have concluded from similar observations on several different samples that purified collagenase breaks down Type 1 and Type 2 collagen and destroys the electron microscopic appearance of the protein polysaccharides of the matrix as well. On the other hand, chymopapain

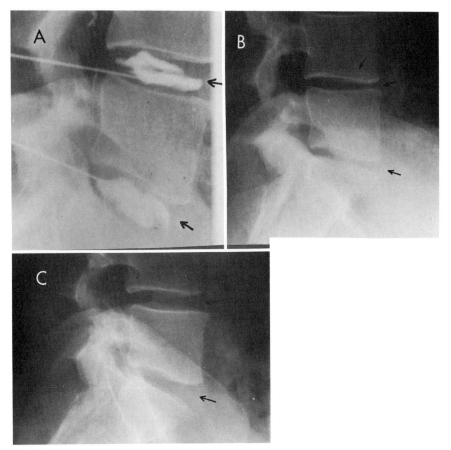

Fig 8–2.—Lateral roentgenograms of lumbar spine in a 24-year-old male. **A,** discogram of fourth and fifth lumbar discs on the day of chymopapain injection. **B,** 60 days after injection. Note narrowing of both discs. **C,** 3 years later, disc heights have been partially restored. (Courtesy L.L. Wiltse.[3] Reprinted by permission of Churchill Livingston, Inc.)

breaks down the proteoglycans but does not disturb the morphologic appearance of the Type 1 and Type 2 collagen fibers on electron microscopy.

DISC HEIGHT AFTER CHEMONUCLEOLYSIS

Leon Wiltse[3] observed eventual restoration of disc height after long-term follow-up of roentgenograms of lumbar discs that had narrowed after chymopapain injection (Fig 8–2). From his observation, we have concluded that chymopapain does not destroy the cellular function of the disc, which can still restore the tissue matrix molecules. An analogous situation occurs in peripheral joint infections caused by certain bacteria that deplete the protein polysaccharide matrix of the articular cartilage without destroying the collagen arcades (e.g., *N. gonorrhea* pyogenic arthritis). The joint space will initially narrow but eventually will be restored.

The disc space narrowing that follows collagenase injection may be irreversible, if we can extrapolate from what we know about the irreversible loss of joint space after peripheral joint infection by bacteria with collagenolytic activity when the collagen arcades have been destroyed. Once the collagen matrix has been destroyed in the disc, the remaining chondrocytes have no scaffolding on which to build a new proteoglycan matrix. Thus far, on long-term follow-up after collagenase injection, Bromley has not observed any restoration of disc height. The speculation that none will be seen after collagenase injection is supported by transmission electron microscopy observations of nucleus pulposus described above, where the morphology of the entire disc matrix is destroyed.

DISCOLYSIS FOLLOWED BY CAT SCANNING

An objective observation of the effectiveness of discolysis with collagenase has been made by C. Gene Coin (Fig 8–3). Using serial com-

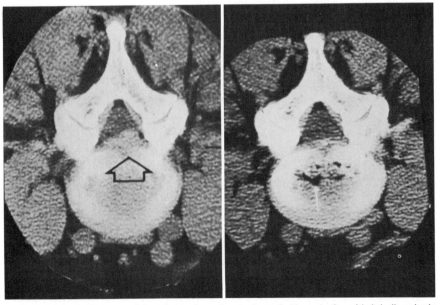

Fig 8–3.—CAT scan of fourth lumbar disc before *(left)* and after *(right)* discolysis with collagenase. Note the disappearance of the herniated disc and gas shadow in the disc space following discolysis. (Courtesy of C. Gene Coin.)

puter-assisted tomography scans before and after chemonucleolysis with collagenase, Coin et al.[4] showed lysis of the herniated portion of the disc, as well as resorption of the nucleus pulposus. A vacuum phenomenon (gas space) actually is produced in the center of the disc and throughout areas of the herniation in some patients. The annulus fibrosus appears to be unaffected. Coin et al. have also found a reduction in ectopic calcification of herniated discs following collagenase injection.

McCulloch[5] noted that some defects persisted after chemonucleolysis with chymopapain on repeat CAT scanning, despite a successful clinical result. He found that the optimum time for repeat CAT scanning after chemonucleolysis was between 3 months and 1 year.

Heithoff[6] noted a consistent shrinkage of the defect in patients who received chymopapain and no defect shrinkage in patients who received an intradiscal saline injection.

Martins and associates[7] performed repeat myelograms after chemonucleolysis with chymopapain and found some patients with persistent extradural defects and others in whom the disc herniation had disappeared.

Relief of sciatica without disappearance of the myelographic defect or CAT scan evidence of disc herniation after chemonucleolysis with chymopapain or collagenase can be explained physiochemically. The theoretical swelling pressure of intact protein polysaccharide may be quite high,[8] and the swelling pressure that this molecule exerts on the nucleus pulposus matrix is limited by the internal restraints of the randomly dispersed and binding collagen fibers of the disc.[9] If the disc protrudes into the spinal canal through an annular tear, the nucleus pulposus may expand with swelling pressures, which have been calculated at more than 300 mm Hg.[10] After chymopapain injection, the swelling pressure of the nucleus pulposus decreases dramatically within the first few hours because of depolymerization of the protein polysaccharides. The disc defect does not have to resolve in order to decompress the nerve and relieve leg pain as long as the swelling pressure is lowered.

Collagenase may theoretically release the internal constraint for swelling of the proteoglycans in the nucleus pulposus by destroying the collagen fibers. If this theory is true, one might expect an initial increase in swelling pressure of the nucleus pulposus following collagenase injection. Subsequent diffusion of the disassociated proteoglycans would lead to eventual decrease in swelling pressure of the disc.

POSTINJECTION PAIN COMPLAINTS

My experience with postinjection pain complaints of 49 patients following Discase injection and 21 patients following Nucleolysin injection has given me the initial impression that more patients in the latter group suffer an initial increase in leg and back pain, which may be severe and may persist for 1–4 weeks before relief is eventually obtained. These observations confirm the theory that breaking the collagen-binding internal constraints to proteoglycan expansion may increase the swelling pressure of the nucleus pulposus, causing increased nerve root compression and pain. A comparative study of pain complaints after discolysis with chymopapain or collagenase is necessary to substantiate these observations. Also, a comparison of in vitro swelling

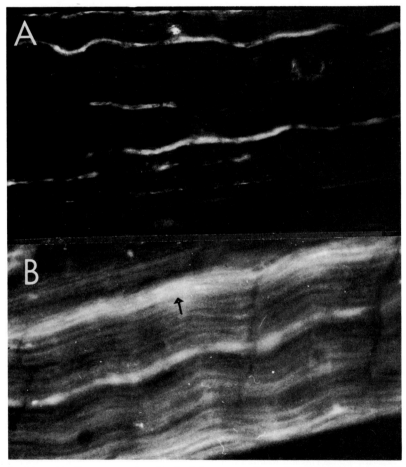

Fig 8–4.—A, fluorescent longitudinal frozen section of rabbit tibial nerve after 2 hours' exposure to 1 ml collagenase (600 units/cc). Note Evan's blue albumin retained within vasa nervorum of nerve fascicles *(white lines)*. **B,** fluorescent longitudinal frozen section opposite tibial nerve; same rabbit as in **A.** Nerve had been exposed to 1 ml chymopapain (4 mg/cc) for 2 hours. Note intravascular Evan's blue albumin has diffused through the microvessels into the intrafascicular space *(black arrow)*.

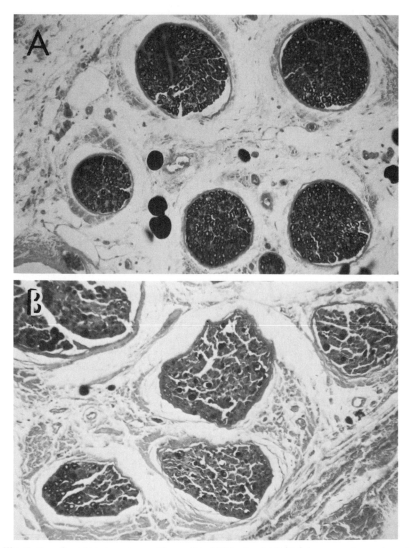

Fig 8–5.—A, microscopic sections ($\times$ 150) of rabbit tibial nerve 4 weeks after exposure to 1 ml collagenase (600 units/cc). Note intact nerve fascicles and slight fibrosis of epineurium. **B,** microscopic section ($\times$ 150) of rabbit tibial nerve 4 weeks after exposure to 1 ml chymopapain (4 mg/cc). Note loss of nerve fibers within the fascicles and fibrosis in the epineurium and endoneurium.

pressures of nucleus pulposus exposed to chymopapain or collagenase should be made.

The injection of collagenase into a large centrally located disc prolapse in the spinal canal may not be as prudent as the use of chymopapain if the above theories are correct.

NEUROTOXICITY

Rydevik et al.[11] determined the effects of therapeutic concentrations of collagenase in the rabbit tibial nerve model previously used to study the effects of chymopapain.[12] Permeability of the intraneural microvessels and the barrier function of the perineural sheath of the rabbit tibial nerve were tested by fluorescent microscopic examination after intravenous infusion or topically applied albumin labeled with Evan's blue. These experiments showed that collagenase solution induced a slight epineural edema and some signs of disruption of the epineurium of the connective tissue stroma of the rabbit tibial nerve. However, the barrier function of the perineural sheath was unaffected, and there were no detectable effects on the permeability of the endoneural microvessels (Fig 8–4). Four to six weeks after exposure, there was no functional impairment of the nerve, but there was minimal evidence of microscopic damage (Fig 8–5). Previous studies by Rydevik et al.[12] with the same model showed that chymopapain had acute effects on the microcirculation, due to disruption of the capillaries of the vasa nervorum. Four to six weeks after exposure to chymopapain, rabbit tibial nerves showed demyelination and diminished functional capacity to transmit impulses. Utilizing this model, it would appear that chymopapain has a deleterious neurotoxic effect when compared to collagenase.

COMPARATIVE ALLERGENICITY

Of 40,000 patients injected with chymopapain, 1% of them, on an average, have been previously sensitized to the enzyme. It is unlikely that this will be the case with collagenase, which is a phylogenetically primitive protein enzyme to which few people have been previously exposed. This enzyme in topically applied burn ointments has produced rare cutaneous allergic reactions. Repeated injections into fibrous bands in patients with Peyronie's disease have failed so far to produce a systemic allergic reaction. However, several thousand patients will have to be injected before a definitive statement can be made concerning the comparative allergenicity of collagenase and chymopapain (see Table 8–1).

INTERACTION OF RADIOPAQUE CONTRAST WITH ENZYMES

Chymopapain

A discogram should precede enzyme injection in order to confirm the diagnosis, level of pathology, and flow pattern of intradiscally injected substances. We studied the interaction of radiopaque contrast dyes with

TABLE 8–2.—Uronic Acid Released (µG/100 MG
Wet Tissue)

AGE	SEX	DISCASE	CONRAY AND DISCASE	DISCASE AND CONRAY
48	M	58	58	58
47	M	58	60	68
40	F	62	52	54
33	F	36	41	32
49	M	28	43	41
28	M	66	72	70
53	M	43	39	41
24	F	21	27	26
35	F	28	25	39
65	M	30	34	39
Mean		43	45	47
Standard error		±54	±4.7	±4.7

chymopapain, using samples of human nucleus pulposus obtained from lumbar spines of cadavers of persons aged 24 to 65. Wet nucleus pulposus tissue (100 mg) was exposed to a solution containing 2 mg of chymopapain at 37 C for 1 hour. Following incubation, the samples were diluted with 10 ml of normal saline, mixed, centrifuged, and the supernatant assayed for uronic acid.

There were no significant differences in uronic acid release from the tissue with Discase alone, the tissue exposed to Conray first and then to Discase, or the tissue exposed to Discase and Conray mixed together and used simultaneously (Table 8–2). If anything, the mixture of Conray and Discase enhanced the release of uronic acids slightly, but not to a significant degree.

Naylor and his colleagues[13] performed a similar study on the effects of radiopaque media on the effect of chymopapain. They determined that the enzymatic action of chymopapain on benzoyl arginine paranitroanilide was actually enhanced by Hypaque, Conray, and Urographin. There was some inhibitory action of metrizamide on chymopapain. They concluded that there was no need to wait between injection of Conray or Hypaque and subsequent enzyme injection with Discase.

In our trials, we did not observe any inhibition of disc space narrowing after Discase injection preceded by a discogram with Conray-60.

Collagenase

We have recently performed similar studies on collagenase (Nucleolysin) to determine the effect of various substances on the action of collagenase on a partially denatured collagen substrate (gelatin) (Table 8–3). Nucleolysin, 600 units per milliliter, was diluted one to one with a 2% gelatin mixture. This mixture was serially diluted with one of the following solutions: a control diluent, serum, Conray-60, cerebrospinal

TABLE 8–3.—GELATINASE ACTIVITY OF COLLAGENASE (600 units/ml)

DILUTION FACTOR	UNITS/ML	SERUM	DILUENT	CONRAY	CSF	0.9%NaCl	XYLOCAINE
1:4	150						
1:8	75.0						
1:16	37.5						
1:32	18.8						
1:64	9.38						
1:128	4.69	○	○				○
1:256	2.34	⊗		○	◑◑		
1:512	1.17	⊗		●		●◑◑	
1:1024	0.586		⊗⊗				
1:2048	0.293						
1:4096	0.146						

Dilution positive experiment no. 1 = ○, 2 = ●, 3 = ◑, 4 = ⊗.
Courtesy of Octavio V. Martinez, Ph.D., Surgical Research Laboratories, University of Miami.

fluid, balanced salt solution, or Xylocaine. The final dilution factor of the collagenase solution was between 1 and 4 and 1 and 4,096. The final concentration of collagenase was 150 units per milliliter in the initial dilution of 1 to 4, and 0.146 units per milliliter in the final dilution.

The samples were incubated for 18 hours at 37 C and then refrigerated. If gelling occurred, the dilution of the collagenase was too high or its action was inhibited by the diluent used. The diluent and balanced salt solution controls did not vary from the various other materials used for serial dilution with respect to the last dilution of collagenase, which prevented gelling by enzyme action on the gelatin. From these results, we concluded that the action of collagenase on gelatin was not inhibited by the substances tested. Although the serum did not inhibit the action of collagenase on gelatin, the dilutional effect did. If this result can be extrapolated to the clinical situation, direct intravascular injection of therapeutic doses of collagenase would be diluted well beyond the threshold determined in this in vitro study.

We have not seen any inhibition of postinjection disc space narrowing after discograms with Conray before collagenase injection. We conclude that it is safe to perform a discogram with Conray-60 before collagenase injection.

COST OF INTRADISCAL THERAPY VERSUS SURGERY

We determined the average length of hospital stay and hospital costs for 10 patients who underwent chemonucleolysis with collagenase, compared with data for 10 patients who underwent surgical disc excisions in 1982 at Jackson Memorial Hospital, University of Miami School of Medicine, Dade County, Florida (Table 8–4). These figures were deter-

TABLE 8–4.—Average Hospital Stay and Average Cost
for Herniated Disc Treatment Methods

PROCEDURE	AVERAGE LENGTH OF HOSPITAL STAY (DAYS)	AVERAGE TOTAL COST
Chemonucleolysis	2.3	$1,549.02
Disc excision	6.6	4,203.21
Myelography and chemonucleolysis	4.3	1,905.48
Myelography and disc excision	9.6	5,427.67

mined from the patients' hospital bills. The average length of stay for a patient undergoing disc injection therapy alone without a myelogram was 2.3 days, and the total average cost was $1,549. The average length of stay and cost for a patient undergoing surgical disc excision was 6.6 days and $4,203. When myelography preceded the injection or surgery, the length of stay and hospital cost were proportionately higher.

According to this data, intradiscal therapy for proved disc displacement requires half the inpatient hospital time and hospital cost. When considering the decreased morbidity and risk as compared to surgery, intradiscal therapy will have an enormous economic impact on cost containment and delivery of health care for patients requiring this treatment.

FDA APPROVAL OF CHYMOPAPAIN

In November 1982, the Food and Drug Administration approved Chymodiactin, a brand of chymopapain produced by Smith Laboratories. In my opinion, it is a matter of time before the FDA approves Discase, Travenol Laboratories' brand of chymopapain, for release. The release of Nucleolysin (collagenase) is anticipated in 1983, if current clinical trials continue to show the presently observed benefits and low risks.

CONCLUSION

Intradiscal therapy for proved disc displacement is a dramatic breakthrough in the treatment of this common disorder that afflicts mankind. As long as the technique is not overused, patients will benefit; and the next edition of this book will not have to contain admonitions concerning failure of therapy due to poor patient selection. Rather, it can concentrate on the development of a better enzyme, incorporating the best features of both chymopapain and collagenase without the adverse side effects of either drug.

REFERENCES

1. Mathews M.B.: The interaction of collagen and acid mucopolysaccharides: A model for connective tissue. *Biochem. J.* 96:710, 1965.
2. Buckwalter J.A.: The fine structure of human intervertebral disc, in White A.A. and Gordon S.L. (eds.): *The American Academy of Orthopaedic Surgeons Symposium on Idiopathic Low Back Pain.* St. Louis, C.V. Mosby Co., 1982.
3. Wiltse L.L.: Chemonucleolysis, in Mickibbin B. (ed.): *Yearbook.* London, Churchill Livingston, Inc., 1983.
4. Coin C.G., Coin J.T., Garrett J.K.: Experimental CT controlled discolysis, in Post M.J.D. (ed.): *Computer Tomography of the Spine.* Baltimore, Williams & Wilkins Co., 1983.
5. McCulloch J.S.: Computed tomography before and after chemonucleolysis, in Post M.J.D. (ed.): *Computer Tomography of the Spine.* Baltimore, Williams & Wilkins Co., 1983.
6. Heithoff K.P.: High resolution computer tomography and stenosis, in Post M.J.D. (ed.): *Computer Tomography of the Spine.* Baltimore, Williams & Wilkins Co., 1983.
7. Martins A.N., Ramirez A., Johnston J., Schwetschenau P.R.: Double-blind evaluation of chemonucleolysis for herniated lumbar discs. Late results. *J. Neurosurg.* 49:816, 1978.
8. Charnley J.: The imbibition of fluid as a cause of herniation of the nucleus pulposus. *Lancet* Jan. 19, p. 1:124, 1952.
9. Woessner J.F., Jr.: Enzymatic mechanisms for the degradation of connective tissue matrix, in Owen P., Godfellow J., Bullough P. (eds.): *Orthopaedics and Traumatology.* London, William Heinemann Medical Books, Ltd., 1980.
10. Hendry N.G.C.: The hydration of the nucleus pulposus and its relation to intervertebral disc derangement. *J. Bone Joint Surg.* 40B:132, 1958.
11. Rydevik B., Brown M., Ehira T., Nordborg C.: Effects of Collagenase on Nerve Tissue. Paper presented to International Society for the Study of the Lumbar Spine, Toronto, June 1982.
12. Rydevik B., Brånemark P.I., Nordborg C., et al.: Effects of chymopapain on nerve tissue. *Spine* 1:137, 1976.
13. Naylor A., Earland C., Robinson J.: The effect of diagnostic radio-opaque fluids used in discography on chymopapain activity. *Spine,* accepted for publication, 1983.

Bibliography

Abadi D.M., Mortvedt D.G.: Inhibition of hydrolysis of chondromucoprotein by plasma proteolytic inhibitor. *Enzyme* 12:41, 1971.

Abbott F.K., Mack M., Wolf S.: The action of banthine on the stomach and duodenum of man: With observations on the effects of placebos. *Gastroenterology* 20:249, 1952.

Abdulla A.F., Ditto E.W., Byrd E.W., et al.: Extreme-lateral lumbar disc herniations. *J. Neurosurg.* 41:229, 1974.

Ackerman W.: Vertebral trephine biopsy. *Ann. Surg.* 143:373, 1956.

Adams R.: Internal-mammary-artery ligation for coronary insufficiency: Evaluation. *N. Engl. J. Med.* 258:113, 1958.

Adams P., Eyre D., Muir H.: Biochemical aspects of development and aging of human lumbar intervertebral discs. *Rheumatol. Rehabil.* 16:22, 1977.

Advance Biofactures Corp.: *Report on the Failure of Nucleolysin Lot #903 to Sensitize Guinea Pigs When Administered Intraperitoneally.* Lynbrook, N.Y., 1979.

Advance Biofactures Corp.: *Clinical Protocol: An Evaluation of the Effects of Intradiscal Collagenase on Herniated Intervertebral Discs.* Lynbrook, N.Y., Revised Apr. 23, 1981.

Advance Biofactures Corp.: *Clinical Protocol for Phase 3: An Evaluation of the Effect of Intradiscal Collagenase on Herniated Intervertebral Lumbar Discs.* Lynbrook, N.Y., Revised Dec. 3, 1981.

Ahmadi J., Segall H., Zee C., et al.: Myelography with metrizamide. *Contemp. Orthopaed.* 4:191, 1981.

American Academy of Orthopedic Surgeons: *Report of the Committee on Chymopapain (Discase).* Chicago, Ill., American Academy of Orthopedic Surgeons, 1975.
[*Dose response data and a compilation of Phase 3 results of the study on chymopapain.*]

American Academy of Orthopedic Surgeons: *A Glossary on Spinal Terminology,* Document 675–80. Chicago, Ill., American Academy of Orthopedic Surgeons, 1980.
[*A good start toward unification of terminology of the spine.*]

American Association of Neurologic Surgeons: Position statement on chymopapain. *J. Neurosurg.* 42:373, 1975.

American Hospital Formulary Service: Sodium iothalamate. *Am. Soc. Hosp. Pharm.* 36:68, 1966.

Anderson K., Berg S.: The relationship between some psychological factors and the outcome of medical rehabilitation. *Scand. J. Rehabil. Med.* 7:166, 1975.

Apfelback H.: Current status of Discase. Read before the American Academy of Orthopedic Surgeons, Las Vegas, Feb. 1977.

Apfelback H.W., Fossier C.H.: Chemonucleolysis: A salvage procedure in the "failed" laminectomy. Read before the American Association of Orthopedic Surgeons, San Francisco, Feb. 1974.

Apfelback H.W., Jacobs R.S., Ray R.D.: Chemonucleolysis in the treatment of low back pain and sciatica. *Surg. Clin. North Am.* 55:181, 1975.

Armstrong J.R.: *Lumbar Disc Lesions: Pathogenesis and Treatment of Low Back Pain Sciatica.* Baltimore, Williams & Wilkins Co., 1965.

Armstrong J.R.: The causes of unsatisfactory results from the operative treatments of lumbar disc lesions. *J. Bone Joint Surg.* 33-B:31, 1951.

Arnell S.: Myelography with water-soluble contrast. *Acta Radiol. [Suppl.] (Stockh.)* 75, 1948.

Arnon R., Shapira E.: Comparison between the antigenic structure of mutually related enzymes: Study with papain and chymopapain. *Biochemistry* 7:4196, 1968.

Aussman R.K.: Personal communication, 1974.

Backache and sciatica: A new breakthrough or a new controversy? *Med. J. Aust.* 1:3, 1974.

Badgley C.E.: The articular facets in relation to low-back pain and sciatica radiation. *J. Bone Joint Surg.* 23:481, 1941.

Ball E.J.: A new treatment of ganglion. *Am. J. Surg.* 50:722, 1940.

Ball J.: Enthesopathy of rheumatoid and ankylosing spondylitis. *Ann. Rheum. Dis.* 30:213, 1971.
[*Reviews pathophysiology and differential diagnosis of rheumatoid spondylitis.*]

Balls A.K., Lineweaver H.: Isolation and properties of crystalline papain. *J. Biol. Chem.* 130:669, 1939.

Barash H.L., Galante J.O., Lambert C.N., et al.: Spondylolisthesis and tight hamstrings. *J. Bone Joint Surg.* 52-A:1319, 1970.

Barr J.S.: "Sciatica" caused by intervertebral disc lesions: A report of forty cases of rupture of the intervertebral disc lesions, occurring in the low lumbar spine and causing pressure on the cauda equina. *J. Bone Joint Surg.* 19:323, 1937.
[*One of the earliest clinical studies on surgical treatment for disc displacement.*]

Barr J.S.: Ruptured intervertebral disc and sciatic pain. *J. Bone Joint Surg.* 29:429, 1947.

Barr J.S.: Low-back and sciatic pain: Results of treatment. *J. Bone Joint Surg.* 33-A:663, 1951.

Barr J.S., Hampton A.O., Mixter W.J.: Pain low in the back and "sciatica" due to lesions of the intervertebral disks. *JAMA* 109:1265, 1937.

Barr J.S., Kubik C.S., Molloy M.K., et al.: Evaluation of and results in the treatment of ruptured lumbar intervertebral discs with protrusion of nucleus pulposus. *Surg. Gynecol. Obstet.* 125:1, 1967.

Barr J.S., Mixter W.J.: Posterior protrusion of the lumbar intervertebral discs. *J. Bone Joint Surg.* 23:444, 1941.

Barrett A.J., Starkey P.M.: The interaction of α_2-macroglobulin with proteases. *Biochem. J.* 133:709, 1973.
[*Documents the basis for assuming that enzymes are inactivated when they are inadvertently injected intravascularly.*]

Barry P., Hume Kendall P.: Cortico-steroid infiltration of the extradural space. *Ann. Phys. Med.* 6:267, 1962.

Battle over chymopapain rages on. *Med. World News* 17:26, 1976.

Batts M. Jr.: Rupture of the nucleus pulposus: An anatomical study. *J. Bone Joint Surg.* 21:121, 1939.

Bauer D. deF.: *Lumbar Discography and Low Back Pain.* Springfield, Ill., Charles C Thomas, Publisher, 1960.

Bauman G.I.: The cause and treatment of certain types of low back pain and sciatica. *J. Bone Joint Surg.* 6:909, 1924.

Baxter Laboratories: *Chymopapain.* Research summary prepared by the Scientific Services Section, Research and Development Dept., Morton Grove, Ill., June 1963, pp. 1–17.

Baxter Laboratories: *Annual Report to Stockholders.* Morton Grove, Ill., 1975, p. 5.

Baxter-Travenol Laboratories: *Protocol for the Double Blind Study Comparing Discase to Placebo.* Morton Grove, Ill. 1974.

Baxter-Travenol Laboratories: *Protocol for Double-Blind Investigation of C.E.I. Injection vs. Saline in Clinical Trials.* Morton Grove, Ill., Feb. 1977.

Bazerque P.M., Galmarini J.C., Evangelista J.C.: Double blind test on the anti-inflammatory effect of proteolytic enzymes. *Medicina* 32:357, 1972.

Beals R.K., Hickman N.W.: Industrial injuries of the back and extremities: Comprehensive evaluation—An aid in prognosis and management. A study on one hundred and eighty patients. *J. Bone Joint Surg.* 54-A:1593, 1972.

[Documents the socioeconomic contribution to compensation, pain, and suffering.]

Beatty R.A.: Treatment with chymopapain, letter. *J. Neurosurg.* 39:793, 1973.

Beecher H.K.: Appraisal of drugs intended to alter subjective responses: Symptoms. Report to Council on Pharmacy and Chemistry. *JAMA* 158:399, 1955. *[Discusses the importance of controlled studies for treatments that alter subjective symptoms.]*

Beecher H.K.: Powerful placebo. *JAMA* 159:1602, 1955.

Beecher H.K.: Relationship of significance of wound to pain experienced. *JAMA* 161:1609, 1956.

Beecher H.K.: *Measurement of Subjective Responses: Quantitative Effects of Drugs.* New York, Oxford University Press, 1959.

Beecher H.K.: Surgery as placebo: A quantitative study of bias. *JAMA* 176:1102, 1961.

Bentley G.: Papain-induced degenerative arthritis. *J. Bone Joint Surg.* 53-B:324, 1971.

Bergman M.: A classification of proteolytic enzymes. *Adv. Enzymol.* 2:49, 1942.

Birkland I.W. Jr., Taylor T.K.F.: Vascular injuries in lumbar disc surgery. *Law. Med. J.* 4:45, 1968.

Blair C.R., Roth R.F., Zintel H.A.: Measurement of coronary artery blood flow following experimental ligation of internal mammary artery. *Ann. Surg.* 152:325, 1960.

Blikra G.: Intradural herniated lumbar disc. *J. Neurosurg.* 31:676, 1969.

Bobechko W.P., Hirsch C.: Autoimmune response to nucleus pulposus in the rabbit. *J. Bone Joint Surg.* 47-B:574, 1965. *[Raises the question; does an autoimmune response to nucleus pulposus occur?]*

Borski S.S., Smith R.A.: Ureteral injury in lumbar disc operation. *J. Neurosurg.* 17:925, 1960.

Bouillet R.: Treatment of low back pain and sciatica by intradiskal injection of chymopapain. *Acta Orthop. Belg.* 42:146, 1976.

Bradford F.K.: Certain anatomic and physiologic aspects of the intervertebral disc. *South. Surg.* 10:623, 1941.

Bradford F.K., Spurling R.G.: *The Intervertebral Disc: With Special Reference to Rupture of the Annulus Fibrosus With Herniation of the Nucleus Pulposus.* Springfield, Ill., Charles C Thomas, Publisher, 1941, p. 158.

Brånemark P.-I.: Tissue effects of chymopapain, letter. *J. Neurosurg.* 42:488, 1975.

Brånemark P.-I.; Ekholm R., Lumdskog J:, et al.: Tissue response to chymopapain in different concentrations: Animal investigations on microvascular effects. *Clin Orthop.* 67:52, 1969.
[*Demonstration of the mechanism of tissue toxicity from chymopapain through microvascular injury.*]

Brill I.C., et al.: Internal mammary ligation. *Northwest Med.* 5:483, 1958.

Still dissolving discs? *Br. Med. J.* 2:1107, 1977.

Bromley J.: Intervertebral discolysis with collagenase. Read before the International Society for the Study of the Lumbar Spine, Paris, June 1981.

Bromley J.: Personal communication, 1982.

Bromley J., Gomez J.: Lumbar intervertebral discolysis with collagenase. *Spine,* in press.
[*Data from the original clinical trial with collagenase.*]

Bromley J., Hirst J., Osman M., et al.: Collagenase: An experimental study of intervertebral disc dissolution. *Spine* 5:126, 1980.
[*Pharmacology and toxicology of collagenase.*]

Bromely J., Santaro A., Cohen P., et al.: Double-blind evaluation of collagenase injection for herniated lumbar discs. Read before the Deidesheimes Gespräch, Deidesheim, Germany, May 1982.
[*The prospective placebo-controlled study of collagenase.*]

Brown J.E.: The enzyme dissolution of intervertebral disk by the use of chymopapain. *Clin. Orthop.* 38:193, 1965.

Brown J.E.: A case post hoc, ergo propter hoc: Addendum or rebuttal for the symposium on chemonucleolysis. Read before the Association of Bone and Joint Surgeons, San Diego, Calif., 1968.

Brown J.E.: Clinical studies on chemonucleolysis. *Clin. Orthop.* 67:94, 1969.

Brown M.D.: *The Pathophysiology of the Intervertebral Disc,* thesis. Philadelphia, Thomas Jefferson University, 1969.

Brown M.D.: The pathophysiology of the intervertebral disc. *Orthop. Clin. North Am.* 2:359, 1971.

Brown M.D.: The diagnosis of back pain syndromes. *Orthop. Clin. North Am.* 6:233, 1975.

Brown M.D.: Chemonucleolysis with Discase: Technique, results, case reports. *Spine* 1:115, 1976.
[*Describes the technique and compares the benefits and risks of chemonucleolysis versus surgery.*]

Brown M.D.: Low back strain and rupture of the intervertebral disc: Section 2—Diagnosis of back pain syndromes; Section 4—Treatment of painful back syndromes, in *Practice of Orthopaedic Surgery,* ed. 2. Hagerstown, Md., Harper & Row, 1977, chap. 14.

Brown M.D.: Lumbar spine fusion, in Finneson B.E. (ed.): *Low Back Pain,* ed. 2. Philadelphia, J.B. Lippincott Co., 1979, chap. 11.
[*A good description of the symptoms and signs differentiating mechanical insufficiency from degenerative disc disease.*]

Brown M.D.: Recent advances in diagnosis and surgery for painful spinal disorders. *J. Fla. Med. Assoc.* 66:63, 1979.

Brown M.D.: *Report to Baxter-Travenol of the Long-Term (4-year) Telephone Follow-up of the Double-Blind Study.* 1981.

Brown M.D.: Spinal surgery: Current status of chemonucleolysis. Lecture, University of Miami School of Medicine, Miami Beach, Fla., April 1981.

Brown M.D.: Revision spine surgery: A second opinion. Lecture, University of Miami School of Medicine, Miami Beach, Fla., April 1982.

Brown M.D., Daroff R.B.: The double blind study comparing Discase to placebo: An editorial comment. *Spine* 2:233, 1977.
[*Flaws in the original double-blind study of chymopapain are clearly defined.*]

Brown M.D., Panjabi M., Lindahl S., et al.: Measurement of disc degeneration by simultaneous volume and pressure recordings during discography. Read before the International Society for the Study of the Lumbar Spine, Toronto, June 1982.
[*Flow patterns of intradiscally injected substances in degenerative disc disease.*]

Brown M.D., Ramos M.: In vitro effects of chymopapain, iothalamate and EDTA on nucleus pulposus. Lecture, University of Miami School of Medicine, Miami Beach, Fla., August 1980.

Brown M.D., Rydevik B.: Effects of collagenase on nerve tissue. Read before the Deidesheimes Gespräch, Deidesheim, Germany, May 1982.

Brown M.D., Tsaltas T.T.: Studies on the permeability of the intervertebral disc during skeletal maturation. *Spine* 1:240, 1976.

Bryant J.H., Leder I.G., Stetlen D. Jr.: The release of chondroitin sulfate from rabbit cartilage following the intravenous injection of crude papain. *Arch. Biochem.* 76:122, 1958.
[*Describes the mechanism of action of crude papain.*]

Buckwalter J.A.: The fine structure of human intervertebral disc, in White A.A., Gordon S.L. (eds.): *American Academy of Orthopedic Surgeons Symposium on Idiopathic Low Back Pain.* St. Louis, C.V. Mosby Co., 1982, chap. 9.
[*An excellent description of the fine structure of the intervertebral disc.*]

Calvé J., Galland M.: The intervertebral nucleus pulposus: Its anatomy, its physiology, its pathology. *J. Bone Joint Surg.* 12:555, 1930.

Carruthers C.D., Kousaie K.N.: Surgical treatment after chemonucleolysis failure. *Clin. Orthop.* 165:172, 1982.

Cayle T., Lopez-Ramos B.: Some properties of chymopapain, abstracted, in *140th Meeting of the American Chemical Society of Chicago,* 1961, p. 190.

Cayle T., Saletan L.T., Lopez-Ramos B.: Some papain fractions and their characteristics. *Proc. Am. Soc. Brew. Chem.,* 1964, pp. 142–153.

Charnley J.: The imbibition of fluid as a cause of herniation of the nucleus pulposus. *Lancet* 124, 1952.
[*The classic early study explaining the pathophysiology of nerve injury from disc displacement.*]

Chemonucleolysis: Better than laminectomy? *JAMA* 224:287, 1973.

Chemonucleolysis. *Lancet* 1:1022, 1975.

Choudhury A.R., Taylor J.C.: Cauda equina syndrome in lumbar disc disease. *Acta Orthop. Scand.* 51:493, 1980.
[*Important for differential diagnosis of contraindications to intradiscal therapy.*]

Chudnovskii N.A.: The dissolution of a prolapsed intervertebral disc with the proteolytic enzyme papain in experimental conditions. *Eksp. Khir. Anest.* 11:46, 1966.

Chymopapain: A case study in federal drug regulation. *JAMA* 240:203, 1978.

Chymopapain: Licensure is near. *Med. World News* 15:6, 1974.

Chymopapain and the intervertebral disc. *Lancet* 2:815, 1967.

Chymopapain pulled off IND status. *Med. World News* 16:38, 1975.

Chrisman O.D.: Biochemical aspects of degenerative joint disease. *Clin. Orthop.* 64:77, 1969.

Chrisman O.D., Mittnacht A., Snook G.A.: A study of the results following rotary manipulation in a lumbar intervertebral disc syndrome. *J. Bone Joint Surg.* 43-B:43, 1964.
[*An early controlled study of disc displacement.*]

Clagett J., Tokuda S., Englehard W.: Chymopapain C, on immuno-suppressive protease: 1. Partial purification and characterization (37991). *Proc. Soc. Exp. Biol. Med.* 145:1250, 1974.

Clark K., Williams P.E., Willis W., et al.: Injection injury of the sciatic nerve. *Clin. Neurosurg.* 17:111, 1970.

Clark M.: Memorandum of an FDA conference on IND 1004 (chymopapain), Nov. 17, 1975.

Clark M.A.: Statement from the Office of Scientific Evaluation, U.S. Food and Drug Administration: Position statement on chymopapain. *J. Neurosurg.* 42:373, 1975.

Cloud G.A., Doyle J.E., Sanford R.L., et al.: *Final Statistical Analysis of the Discase Double Blind Clinical Trial.* Deerfield, Ill., Travenol Laboratories, Biostatistical Services Dept., 1976.
[*A complete statistical analysis of the original double-blind study of chymopapain.*]

Cloward R.B., Buzaid L.L.: Discography: technique, indications and evaluation of normal and abnormal intervertebral disc. *AJR* 68:552, 1952.

Clymer G., Mixter W.J., Voella H.: Experience with spinal cord tumors during the past ten years. *Arch. Neurol. Psychiatry* 5:213, 1921.

Cobb L.S., Thomas G., Dillard D., et al.: Evaluation of internal-mammary-artery ligation by double-blind technic. *N. Engl. J. Med.* 260:1115, 1959.
[*A classic controlled study of surgical treatment for a subjective symptom complex.*]

Cogan J., Symones H., Gibbs D.: Intracapsular cataract extraction using alpha-chymotrypsin. *Br. J. Ophthalmol.* 45:193, 1959.

Coin C.G., Coin J.T., Garrett J.K.: Experimental CT controlled discolysis, in Post M.J.D. (ed.): *Computer Tomography of the Spine.* Baltimore, Williams & Wilkins, 1983, chap. 27.

Collis J.S., Gardiner W.J.: Lumbar discography: An analysis of one thousand cases. *J. Neurosurg.* 19:452, 1962.

Collis J.S.: *Lumbar Discography.* Springfield, Ill., Charles C Thomas, Publisher, 1963.

Colonna P.C., Friedenberg Z.B.: The disc syndrome: Results of the conservative care of patients with positive myelograms. *J. Bone Joint Surg.* 31-A:614, 1949.
[*Data on the natural history of symptomatic disc displacement.*]

Compere E.L., Keyes D.C.: Roentgenological studies of the intervertebral disc. *AJR* 29:774, 1933.

Connolly R.C.: Chemonucleolysis, editorial. *J. Bone Joint Surg.* 59-B:1, 1977.

Coventry M.B.: Low back and sciatic pain: Introduction to symposium, including anatomy, physiology and epidemiology. *J. Bone Joint Surg.* 50-A:167, 1968.

Coventry M.B., Ghormley R.K., Kernohan J.W.: The intervertebral disc: Its microscopic anatomy and pathology. *J. Bone Joint Surg.* 27:105, 233, 460, 1945.
[*A complete review of the anatomy and pathology of the intervertebral disc.*]

Craig F.S.: Vertebral body biopsy. *J. Bone Joint Surg.* 38-A:93, 1956.

Craig W.M., Walsh M.N.: Diagnosis and treatment of low back and sciatic pain caused by protruded intervertebral disk and hypertrophied ligaments. *Minn. Med.* 22:511, 1939.

Craig W.M., Walsh M.N.: Neuro-anatomical and physiological aspects and significance of sciatica. *J. Bone Joint Surg.* 23:417, 1941.

Crawford A.S., Mitchell C.L., Granger G.R.: Surgical treatment of low back pain with sciatic radiation: Preliminary report on 346 cases. *Arch. Surg.* 59:724, 1949.

Criep L., Beam L.: Allergy to trypsin. *J. Allergy* 35:425, 1964.

Crout J.R.: Statement from the Bureau of Drugs, U.S. Food and Drug Administration. *J. Neurosurg.* 42:373, 1975.

Dabezies E.J., Brunet M.: Chemonucleolysis vs. laminectomy. *Orthopedics* 1:26, 1978.

Dandy W.E.: Loose cartilage from intervertebral disk simulating tumor of the spinal cord. *Arch. Surg.* 19:660, 1929.

Dandy W.E.: Recent advances in the diagnosis and treatment of ruptured intervertebral discs. *Am. Surg.* 115:514, 1942.

Danforth M.S., Wilson P.D.: The anatomy of the lumbosacral region in relation to sciatic pain. *J. Bone Joint Surg.* 7:109, 1925.

Davidson E.W., Woodhall B.: Biochemical alterations in herniated intervertebral disks. *J. Biol. Chem.* 234:2951, 1959.

Day P.L.: Lateral approach for lumbar diskogram and chemonucleolysis. *Clin. Orthop.* 67:90, 1969.

Day P.L.: Early, interim, and long term observations on chemonucleolysis in 876 patients: With special comments on the lateral approach. *Clin. Orthop.* 99:64, 1974.

Déjerine J.: Sur la claudication intermittente de la moelle epinière. *Rev. Neurol.* 14:341, 1906.

Delage C., Irey N.: Anaphylactic deaths: A clinicopathologic study of 43 cases. *J. Forensic Sci.* 17:525, 1972.

DePalma A.F., Rothman R.H.: Surgery of the lumbar spine. *Clin. Orthop.* 63:162, 1969.

DeSaussure R.L.: Vascular injury coincident to disc surgery. *J. Neurosurg.* 16:222, 1959.

Deucher W.G., Love J.G.: Pathologic aspects of posterior protrusions of the intervertebral disks. *Arch. Pathol.* 27:201, 1939.

Dickson I.R., Happey F., Pearson C.H., et al.: Decrease in hydrothermal stability of collagen on aging in the human intervertebral disk. *Nature* 215:50, 1967.

Dickson I.R., Happey F., Pearson C.H.: Variations in the protein components of human intervertebral disk with age. *Nature* 215:52, 1967.

Digby J.M., Kersley J.B.: Pyogenic non-tuberculous spinal infection. *J. Bone Joint Surg.* 61-B:47, 1979.

[*A current review of the diagnosis and treatment of disc space infection.*]

Dilke T.F.W., Burry H.C., Grahame R.: Extradural corticosteriod injection in management of lumbar nerve root compression. *Br. Med. J.* 2:635, 1973.

DiMaio V.J.: Two anaphylactic deaths after chemonucleolysis. *J. Forensic Sci.* 21:187, 1976.

Dimond E.G., Kittle C.F., Crockett J.E.: Evaluation of internal mammary artery ligation and sham procedure in angina pectoris. *Circulation* 18:712, 1958.

DiSalve J., Schubert M.: Interaction during fibril formation of soluble collagen with cartilage protein polysaccharide. *Biopolymers* 4:247, 1966.

DiSalve J., Schubert M.: Specific interactions of some cartilage protein-polysaccharides with freshly precipitating calcium phosphate. *J. Biol. Chem.* 242:705, 1967.

Doenicke A., Lorenz W.: Histamine release in anesthesia and surgery: Premedication with H_1- and H_2-receptor antagonists—Indications, benefits and possible problems. *Klin. Wochenschr.* 60:1039, 1982.

Donohue W.L.: Pathology of the intervertebral disc. *Am. J. Med. Sci.* 198:419, 1939.

Doroshow L.W., Young Y.M., Robbins M.A.: Intrathecal injection: an unusual complication of translumbar aortography—Case report. *J. Urol.* 88:438, 1962.

Dubuc F., Rouleau C.: Lumbo-sciatica and chemonucleolysis. *Union Med. Can.* 106:65, 1977.

Dunn J.E., Johnson C.L., Cox W.: Treatment of lumbar disks with chymopapain. *Phys. Ther.* 56:399, 1976.

Eastoe J.E., Courts A.: *Practical Analytical Methods for Connective Tissue Proteins.* Springfield, Charles C Thomas, Publisher, 1964, p. 39.

Ebata M., Takahashi Y.: Proteolytic specificity of chymopapain: Hydrolysis of the fraction B of oxidized insulin. *Biochim. Biophys. Acta* 118:210, 1966.

Ebata M., Tsunoda J., Yasunobu K.T.: Changes in the conformation of chymopapain during the activation process. *Biochem. Biophys. Res. Commun.* 22:445, 1966.

Ebata M., Tsunoda J., Yasunobu K.T.: Effects of diisopropylphosphorofluoridate on papain, chymopapain and bromelain. *Biochem. Biophys. Res. Commun.* 9:173, 1962.

Ebata M., Yasunobu K.T.: Chymopapain: I. Isolation, crystallization and preliminary characterization. *J. Biol. Chem.* 237:1086, 1962.

Ebata M., Yasunobu K.T.: Chymopapain: III. The inhibition of chymopapain by diisopropylphosphorofluoridate. *Biochim. Biophys. Acta* 73:132, 1963.

Echols D.H.: Surgical treatment of sciatica: Results 3 to 8 years after operation. *Arch. Neurol. Psychiatry* 61:672, 1949.

Echols D.H.: Sensory rhizotomy following operation for ruptured disc. *J. Neurosurg.* 31:335, 1969.

Eder J., Arnon R.: Structural and functional comparison of antibodies to common and specific determinants of papain and chymopapain. *Immunochemistry* 10:535, 1973.

Edholm P., Fernström I., Lindblom K.: Extradural lumbar disk puncture. *Acta Radiol. [Diagn.] (Stockh.)* 6:322, 1967.
[*The original description of the lateral extradural approach to lumbar intervertebral disc.*]

Eie N.: Load capacity of the low back. *J. Oslo City Hosp.* 16:4, 1966.

Eie N., Kristiansen K.: Complications and hazards of traction in the treatment of ruptured lumbar intervertebral disks. *J. Oslo City Hosp.* 12:5, 1962.

Einbinder J., Schubert M.: Binding of mucopolysaccharides and dyes by collagen. *J. Biol. Chem.* 188:335, 1951.

Elsberg C.A.: Experiences in spinal surgery: Observations upon 60 laminectomies for spinal disease. *Surg. Gynecol. Obstet.* 16:117, 1913.

Engel G.L.: "Psychogenic" pain and pain-prone patient. *Am. J. Med.* 26:899, 1959.
[*An excellent description of the pain-prone patient.*]

Engfeldt B., Hulth A., Westerborn C.: Effect of papain on bone: I. Histologic autoradiographic and microradiographic study on young dogs. *Arch. Pathol. Lab. Med.* 68:600, 1959.

Erlacher P.R.: Nucleography. *J. Bone Joint Surg.* 34-B:204, 1952.

Evans C.: Chemonucleolysis. *Nurs. Times* 71:1539, 1975.

Evans F.G., Lissner H.R.: Strength of intervertebral discs, abstracted. *J. Bone Joint Surg.* 36-A:185, 1954.

Evans W.: Intrasacral epidural injection in the treatment of sciatica. *Lancet* 2:1225, 1930.

Eyre D., Muir H.: Quantitative analysis of types I and II collagens in human intervertebral discs at various ages. *Biochim. Biophys. Acta* 492:29, 1977.

Eyring E.J.: Biochemistry and physiology of the intervertebral disc. *Clin. Orthop.* 67:16, 1969.

Ehrlich M.G., Mankin H.J., Treadwell B.V.: Acid hydrolase activity in osteoarthritic and normal human cartilage. *J. Bone Joint Surg.* 55-A:1068, 1973.

Farrell B.P., MacCracken W.B.: Spine fusion for protruding intervertebral disc. *J. Bone Joint Surg.* 23:457, 1941.

Feffer H.L.: Treatment of low back and sciatic pain by the injection of hydrocortisone into degenerated intervertebral discs. *J. Bone Joint Surg.* 38-A:585, 1956.
[*A classic clinical study using hydrocortisone for intradiscal therapy.*]

Feffer H.L.: Therapeutic intradiscal hydrocortisone: A long term study. *Clin. Orthop.* 6:100, 1969.

Feffer H.L.: Transcript of proceedings, Subcommittee on Health of the Committee on Labor and Public Welfare, Subcommittee on Administrative Practice and Procedure of the Committee on Judiciary. Investigation into the Food and Drug Administration, portion relating to Discase. Washington, D.C., 1974, p. 95.

Feffer H.L., Rizzoli H.V.: Negative myelogram and nucleography. *Postgrad. Med. J.* 19:363, 1956.

Feinberg S.B.: The place of diskography in radiology as based on 2,320 cases. *AJR* 92:1275, 1964.

Felleroni A.E.: Treatment of allergic emergencies. *Mod. Treat.* 5:782, 1968.

Ferrara A., Fenke S., Grieco M., et al.: Anaphylactic reactions to aqueous chymotrypsin. *J. Allergy* 34:460, 1963.

Fessel J.M., Chrisman O.D.: Enzymatic degradation of chondromucoprotein by cell-free extracts of human cartilage. *Arthritis Rheum.* 7:398, 1964.

Fernstrom U.: A discographical study of ruptured lumbar intervertebral discs. *Acta Chir. Scand. Suppl.* 258, 1960.

Finnegan W.J., Fenlin J.M., Marvel J.P., et al.: Results of surgical intervention in the symptomatic multiply-operated back patient. *J. Bone Joint Surg.* 61-A:1077, 1979.

Fish R.G., Crymes T.P., Lovell M.G.: Internal-mammary-artery ligation for angina pectoris: Its failure to produce relief. *N. Engl. J. Med.* 259:418, 1958.

Fisher H.W., Doust V.L.: An evaluation of pretesting in the problem of serious and fatal reactions to excretory venography. *Radiology* 103:497, 1972.

Flint Laboratories: *Chymopapain Injection: A Research Summary.* Morton Grove, Ill., Flint Laboratories, 1964, pp. 1–24.

Foerster O.: The dermatomes in man. *Brain* 56:1, 1933.

Ford L.: Clinical use of chymopapain in lumbar and dorsal disk lesions: An end-result study. *Clin. Orthop.* 67:81, 1969.

Ford L.T.: Experimental study of chymopapain in cats. *Clin. Orthop.* 67:68, 1969.

[An animal study that demonstrated no adverse effect of chymopapain in the epidural space.]

Ford L.T.: Chemonucleolysis. Read before the American Association of Orthopedic Surgeons, Las Vegas, Feb. 1973.

Ford L.T.: Chymopapain: Past, present and future? *Clin. Orthop.* 122:367, 1977.

Ford L.T.: Chymopapain (Discase) for chemonucleolysis for lumbar disc disease in the United States. *Orthop. Rev.* 7:25, 1978.

Ford L.T., Gilula L.A., Murphy W.A., et al.: Analysis of gas in vacuum lumbar disc. *AJR* 128:1056, 1977.

Fordyce W.E.: Operant conditioning as a treatment method in management of selected chronic pain problems. *Northwest Med.* 69:580, 1970.

Fox A.M.: Anaphylactoid shock induced by oral penicillin and resulting in Gerstmann's syndrome. *Br. Med. J.* 2:206, 1965.

Franklin L., Hull E.W.: Lipid content of the intervertebral disc. *Clin. Chem.* 12:5, 1966.

Frantzen E., Zacharie L.: The effect of conservative treatment of lumbago-sciatica. *Nord. Med.* 62:1509, 1959.

Fraser R.D.: Chymopapain for the treatment of intervertebral disc prolapse: A double-blind study. Read before the International Society for the Study of the Lumbar Spine, Toronto, June 1982.
[A well-designed double-blind study of chymopapain (Discase) in the treatment of disc displacement.]

French J.D.: Clinical manifestations of lumbar spinal arachnoiditis: A report of thirteen cases. *Surgery* 20:718, 1946.

Friberg S.: Low back and sciatic pain caused by intervertebral disc herniation. *Acta Chir. Scand.* 85 (suppl. 64), 1941.

Friberg S.: Anatomical studies of lumbar disc degeneration. *Acta Orthop. Scand.* 17:224, 1948.

Friberg S., Hirsch C.: On late results of operative treatment for intervertebral disc prolapse in the lumbar region. *Acta Orthop. Scand.* 93:161, 1946.

Friberg S., Hirsch C.: Anatomical and clinical studies on the lumbar disc degeneration. *Acta Orthop. Scand.* 19:222, 1949.

Friberg S., Hult L.: Comparative study of abrodil myelogram and operative findings in low back pain and sciatica. *Acta Orthop. Scand.* 20:303, 1950/51.

Friedman J., Goldner M.A.: Discography in evaluation of lumbar lesions. *Radiology* 65:653, 1955.

Froning E.C.: Chemonucleolysis for the treatment of disabling lumbar herniated nucleus pulposus in the absence of nerve root involvement. Read before the Western Orthopedic Association, San Diego, Calif. Oct. 25, 1973.

Funkquist B.: Thoraco-lumbar disk protrusion with severe cord compression in the dog: I. Clinical and patho-anatomic observations with special reference to the rate of development of the symptoms of motor loss; II. Clinical observations with special reference to the prognosis in conservative treatment; III. Treatment by decompressive laminectomy. *Acta Vet. Scand.* 3:256, 1962.

Galante J.O.: Tensile properties of the human lumbar annulus fibrosus. *Acta Orthop. Scand. [Suppl.]* 100, 1967.

Gama C.: Neuralgic pain wrongly ascribed to posterior hernia of the intervertebral discs. *J. Int. Coll. Surg.* 13:578, 1950.

Garrick J.G., Sullivan C.R.: A technic of performing diskography in dogs. *Mayo Clin. Proc.* 39:270, 1964.

Gartland J.J.: Judgment in lumbar disc surgery. *Orthop. Clin. North Am.* 2:507, 1971.

Garvin P.J.: Toxicity of collagenase: The relation to enzyme therapy of disc herniation. *Clin. Orthop.* 101:286, 1974.

Garvin P.J., Jennings R.B.: Long-term effects of chymopapain on intervertebral disks of dogs. *Clin. Orthop.* 92:281, 1973.

Garvin P.J., Jennings R.B., Smith L., et al.: Chymopapain: A pharmacologic and toxicologic evaluation in experimental animals. *Clin. Orthop.* 41:204, 1965. [*A good review of the pharmacology and toxicology of chymopapain.*]

Garvin P.J., Jennings R.B., Stern I.J.: Enzymatic digestion of the nucleus pulposus: A review of experimental studies with chymopapain. *Orthop. Clin. North Am.* 8:2, 1977.

Gershater R., Holgate R.C.: Lumbar epidural venography in the diagnosis of disc herniations. *AJR* 126:992, 1976.

Gesler R.M.: Pharmacologic properties of chymopapain. *Clin. Orthop.* 67:47, 1969.

Gherini A., Hande D.: Anaphylactic reactions to chymotrypsin. *Calif. Med.* 94:379, 1961.

Ghormley R.K.: Low back pain with special reference to the articular facets, with presentation of an operative procedure. *JAMA* 101:1773, 1933.

Ghormley R.K., Bickel W.H., Dickson D.D.: Study of acute infectious lesions of intervertebral discs. *South Med. J.* 33:347, 1940.

Gold A., Andrews R.F., Manicom R.E.: Treatment of disk lesions of the lumbar spine by intradisk injections of enzymes. *South. Med. J.* 59:1293, 1966.

Goldie I.: Changes observed in the intervertebral disc after discography. *Acta Pathol. Microbiol. Scand.* 42:193, 1958.

Goldie I.: A clinical trial with indomethacin in low back pain and sciatica. *Acta Orthop. Scand.* 39:117, 1968.

Gottschalk L.A.: Psychologic factors in backache. General Practitioner 33:91, 1966.

Grabias S.: The treatment of spinal stenosis. *J. Bone Joint Surg.* 42-A:308, 1980. [*A thorough review of spinal stenosis.*]

Graham C.E.: Intradiscal enzyme for back pain, letter. *Med. J. Aust.* 2:406, 1973.

Graham C.E.: Backache and sciatica: A report of 90 patients treated by intradiscal injection of chymopapain (Discase). *Med. J. Aust.* 1:5, 1974.

Graham C.E.: Chemonucleolysis: A preliminary report on a double blind study comparing chemonucleolysis and intradiscal administration of hydrocortisone in the treatment of backache and sciatica. *Orthop. Clin. North Am.* 6:259, 1975.

Graham C.E.: Chemonucleolysis: A double blind study comparing chemonucleolysis with intradiscal hydrocortisone in the treatment of backache and sciatica. *Clin. Orthop.* 117:179, 1976.
[*Nonstringent patient selection was a major flaw in this controlled study.*]

Green D.M.: Pre-existing conditions, placebo reactions, and "side effects." *Ann. Intern. Med.* 60:255, 1964.

Green L.N.: Dexamethasone in the management of symptoms due to herniated lumbar disc. *J. Neurol. Neurosurg. Psychiatry* 38:1211, 1975.

Greenwald K.A., Tsaltas T.T.: Papain induced chemical changes in adult rabbit cartilage matrix. *Proc. Soc. Exp. Biol. Med.* 117:885, 1964.

Gresham J.L., Miller R.: Evaluation of the lumbar spine by discography and its use in selection of proper treatment of the herniated disc syndrome. *Clin. Orthop.* 67:29, 1969.

Gross J., Lapiere M.: Collagenolytic activity in amphibious tissues: A tissue culture assay. *Proc. Natl. Acad. Sci. USA* 48:1014, 1962.

Gurdjian E.S., Ostrowski A.Z., Hardy W.G.: Results of operative treatment of protruded and ruptured lumbar discs based on 1,176 operative cases with 82 percent follow-up of 3 to 13 years. *J. Neurosurg.* 18:783, 1961.
[*A large surgical series treated for disc displacement, with long-term follow-up.*]

Gurdjian E.S., Webster J.E.: Lumbar herniations of the nucleus pulposus. *Am. J. Surg.* 76:235, 1948.

Gurdjian N.E.S., Webster J.E., Ostrowski A.Z., et al.: Herniated intervertebral discs based on 1,176 operative patients. *J. Trauma* 1:158, 1961.

Hadley L.A.: Boney masses projecting into the spinal canal opposite a break in the neural arch of the fifth lumbar vertebra. *J. Bone Joint Surg.* 37-A:787, 1955.

Hainsworth A.M., Bingham W.: An allergic circulatory collapse following the administration of muscle relaxants. *Anesthesia* 25:105, 1970.

Hakelius A.: Prognosis in sciatica. *Acta Orthop. Scand. [Suppl.]* 129:1, 1970. *[The classic prospective controlled study of the treatment of disc displacement by nonoperative and operative means.]*

Hallen A.: Hexosamine and ester sulphate content of the human nucleus pulposus at different ages. *Acta Chem. Scand.* 12:1869, 1958.

Hallen A.: Extraction of mucopolysaccharides from connective tissue. *Acta Chem. Scand.* 14:1828, 1960.

Hallen A.: The collagen and ground substance of human intervertebral disc at different ages. *Acta Chem. Scand.* 16:705, 1962.

Hampton A.O.: Iodized oil myelography: Use in the diagnosis of rupture of the intervertebral disk into the spinal canal. *Arch. Surg.* 40:444, 1940.

Hampton A.O., Robinson J.M.: The roentgenographic demonstration of rupture of the intervertebral disk into the spinal canal after injection of Lipiodol: With special reference to unilateral lumbar lesions accompanied by low back pain with "sciatic" radiation. *AJR* 36:728, 1936.

Hanashiro P.K., Weil M.H.: Anaphylactic shock in man. *Arch. Intern. Med.* 119:129, 1967.

Hansen H.J.: A pathologic-anatomical study on disc degeneration in dog. *Acta Orthop. Scand. [Suppl.]* 11, 1952.

Hansen J.W.: Postoperative management in lumbar disc protrusion. *Acta Orthop. Scand. [Suppl.]* 71, 1964.

Hanson R.W., Schwartz H., Barker S.B.: Free and fixed glycogen as physiological entities. *Am. J. Physiol.* 198:80, 1960.

Havik L.J.: *Some Psychological Dimensions of Low Back Pain,* thesis. University of Minnesota, 1949.

Harley C.: Extradural corticosteroid infiltration: A follow-up study of 50 cases. *Ann. Phys. Med.* 9:22, 1967.

Harris R.I., MacNab I.: Structural changes in the lumbar intervertebral discs. *J. Bone Joint Surg.* 36-B:304, 1954.

Hart F.D., Strickland D., Cliffe P.: Measurement of spinal mobility. *Ann. Rheum. Dis.* 33:136, 1974.

Hartman J.T. Winnie A.P., Ramaurthy S., et al.: Intradural and extradural corticosteroids for sciatic pain. *Orthop. Rev.* 12:21, 1974.

Hashimoto A., Ludoweig J.J.: The protein polysaccharides from the nucleus pulposus of whale intervertebral discs: Effect of disulfide reducing reagents. *Biochem. J.* 7:2469, 1968.

Hathaway S.R., McKinley J.C.: *The Minnesota Multiphasic Personality Inventory,* rev. ed. New York, The Psychological Corporation, 1951.

Haughton V.M., Eldevik O.P., Magnaes B., et al.: A prospective comparison of computed tomography and myelography in the diagnosis of herniated lumbar discs. *Radiology* 142:103, 1982.
[*An excellent current study on the use of CT in the diagnosis of herniated discs.*]

Hausen H.-J.: A pathologic-anatomical interpretation of disc degeneration in dogs. *Acta Orthop. Scand.* 20:280, 1950.

Hawkes C.H., Roberts G.M.: Neurogenic and vascular claudication. *J. Neurol. Sci.* 38:337, 1978.

Heithoff K.P.: High resolution computer tomography and stenosis (evaluation of causes and cures of failed back syndromes), in Post M.S.D. (ed.): *Computer Tomography of the Spine.* Baltimore, Williams & Wilkins, 1983, chap. 31.

Henderson R.S.: The treatment of lumbar intervertebral disc protrusion. *Br. Med. J.* 2:597, 1952.

Hendry N.G.C.: The imbibition characteristics of normal and abnormal intervertebral discs. *J. Bone Joint Surg.* 37-B:164, 1955.

Hendry N.G.C.: The hydration of the nucleus pulposus and its relation to intervertebral disc derangement. *J. Bone Joint Surg.* 40-B:132, 1958.
[*The classic description of the biomechanics of degenerated discs.*]

Hentzer L.A.: Conservative and operative treatment of disc prolapse: A follow-up examination of 152 patients. *Ugeskr. Laeger* 135:2258, 1973.

Herrick R.B., Daughety J.S., Hoover B.B.: Clinical and electromyographic evaluation after chemonucleolysis for lumbar disk disease. *South. Med. J.* 68:1552, 1975.

Heripret G., Benoist A., DeBurge A., et al.: The treatment of lumbar disc herniation by chemonucleolysis: A report on 120 patients. Read before the International Society for the Study of the Lumbar Spine, Toronto, June 1982.

Hirsch C.: An attempt to diagnose the level of a disc lesion clinically by disc puncture. *Acta Orthop. Scand.* 18:132, 1948.

Hirsch C.: Studies on the mechanism of low back pain. *Acta Orthop. Scand.* 20:261, 1950.

Hirsch C.: Reaction of intervertebral discs to compression forces. *J. Bone Joint Surg.* 37-A:1188, 1955.

Hirsch C.: Studies on the pathology of low back pain. *J. Bone Joint Surg.* 41-B:237, 1959.
[*The first to suggest using a "chondrolytic enzyme" for intradiscal therapy.*]

Hirsch C.: Efficiency of surgery in low back disorders. *J. Bone Joint Surg.* 47-A:991, 1965.

Hirsch C.: Low back pain etiology and pathogenesis. *Applied Therapy* 8:10:857, 1966.

Hirsch C.: Etiology and pathogenesis of low back pain. *Isr. J. Med. Sci.* 2:362, 1966.

Hirsch C.: Macroscopic rheology in collagen material. *J. Biomech.* 1:13, 1968.

Hirsch C.: Letter to Travenol, March 31, 1971.

Hirsch C., Ingelmark B.E., Miller M.: The anatomical basis for low back pain. *Acta Orthop. Scand.* 33:135, 1961.

Hirsch C., Jonsson B., Lewin T.: Low back symptoms in a Swedish female population. *Clin. Orthop.* 63:171, 1969.

Hirsch C., Nachemson A.: New observations on the mechanical behavior of lumbar discs. *Acta Orthop. Scand.* 23:255, 1953.

Hirsch C., Nachemson A.: The reliability of lumbar disc surgery. *Clin. Orthop.* 29:189, 1963.

Hirsch C., Paulson S., Sylven B., et al.: Biophysical and physiological investigations on cartilage and other mesenchymal tissues: IV. Characteristics of human nuclei pulposi during aging. *Acta Orthop. Scand.* 22:175, 1952.

Hirsch C., Schajowicz F.: Studies on structural changes in the lumbar annulus fibrosus. *Acta Orthop. Scand.* 22:184, 1952.

Hirsch C., Snellman O., Sylven B., et al.: Biophysical and physiological investigations on cartilage and other mesenchymal tissues: II. The ultrastructure of bovine and human nuclei pulposi. *J. Bone Joint Surg.* 33-A:333, 1951.

Hitselberger W.E., Witten R.M.: Abnormal myelograms in asymptomatic patients. *J. Neurosurg.* 28:204, 1968.
[*Why one should* not *treat roentgenograms but should treat patients.*]

Hoerlein B.F.: *Canine Neurology: Diagnosis and Treatment.* Philadelphia, W.B. Saunders Co., 1965.

Holmes R., Ross J., Williams E.: Acute anaphylaxis under anesthesia. *Anesthesia* 26:363, 1971.

Holt E.P. Jr.: Fallacy of cervical discography. *JAMA* 188:799, 1964.

Holt E.P.: The question of lumbar discography. *J. Bone Joint Surg.* 50-A:720, 1968.

Holt E.P.: Transcript of proceedings, Subcommittee on Health of the Committee on Labor and Public Welfare, Subcommittee on Administrative Practice and Procedure of the Committee on Judiciary. Investigation into the Food and Drug Administration, portion relating to Disease. Washington, D.C., 1974, p. 105.

Holt E.P.: The question of chemonucleolysis or all you ever suspected about chemonucleolysis but were afraid to ask. *Orthop. Audio. Synopsis* 6:4, 1974.

Holt E.P. Jr.: The question of chemonucleolysis. *Clin. Orthop.* 105:299, 1974.

Hoogmartens M., VanLoon L., Demedts D., et al.: Comparative study of the results obtained with discectomy and chemonucleolysis. *Acta Orthop. Belg.* 42:134, 1976.

Hoover B.B., Caldwell J.W., Drusen E.M., et al.: Value of polyphasic potentials in diagnosis of lumbar root lesions. *Arch. Phys. Med. Rehabil.* 51:546, 1970.

Horal J.: The clinical appearance of low back pain disorders in the city of Gothenburg, Sweden: Comparisons of incapacitated probands with matched controls. *Acta Orthop. Scand. [Suppl.]* 118, 1969.

Horwitz T.: Lesions of the intervertebral disc and ligamentum flavum of lumbar vertebrae: An anatomic study of 75 human cadavers. *Surgery* 6:410, 1939.

Howell I.: Anaphylactic reaction to Chymotrypsin. *JAMA* 175:134, 1961.

Howland W.J., Curry J.L.: Experimental studies of pantopaque arachnoiditis: I. Animal studies. *Radiology* 87:253, 1966.

Howland W.J., Curry J.L., Butler A.K.: Pantopaque arachnoiditis: Experimental study of blood as a potentiating agent. *Radiology* 80:489, 1963.

Hudgins P.W.: The predictive value of myelography in the diagnosis of ruptured lumbar discs. *J. Neurosurg.* 32:152, 1970.
[*Useful data on the predictability of physical findings in the diagnosis of disc displacement.*]

Hudgins W.R.: Lumbar disk disease: Laminectomy vs. chymopapain chemonucleolysis. *JAMA* 234:703, 1975.

Hult L.: The Munkfors investigation. *Acta Orthop. Scand. [Suppl.]* 16, 1954.

Hult L.: Cervical, dorsal and lumbar spinal syndromes. *Acta Orthop. Scand. [Suppl.]* 17, 1954.

Hulth A., Westerborn O.: The effect of crude papain on the epiphyseal cartilage of laboratory animals. *J. Bone Joint Surg.* 41-B:836, 1959.

Huncke B.H., Jabaay G.A., Sullivan R.: Chemonucleolysis: A preliminary report. *Med. Trial Tech. Q.* 20:80, 1973.

Hurst E.W.: Adhesive arachnoiditis and vascular blockage caused by detergents and other chemical irritants: An experimental study. *J. Pathol. Bacteriol.* 70:167, 1955.

Hurteau E.F., Baird W.C., Sinclair E.: Arachnoiditis following the use of iodized oil. *J. Bone Joint Surg.* 36-A:393, 1954.

Hwang K., Ivy A.C.: A review of the literature on the potential therapeutic significance of papain. *Ann. NY Acad. Sci.* 54:161, 1951.

Idsoe O., Guthrie T., Willcox R.R., et al.: Nature and extent of penicillin side-reactions with particular reference to fatalities from anaphylactic shock. *Bull. WHO* 38:159, 1968.

Inman V.T., Saunders J.: Referred pain from skeletal structures. *J. Nerve Ment. Dis.* 99:660, 1944.
[*A classic work for the diagnostician.*]

Jackson H.B., Winkelman R.K., Bickel W.H.: Nerve endings in the human lumbar spinal column and related structures. *J. Bone Joint Surg.* 48-A:1272, 1966.
[*A clear description of nerve supply to the IVD.*]

Jacobi A.: Note on Papayotin. *Therapeutic Gazette* 10:145, 1886.

James L., Austen F.: Total systemic anaphylaxis in man. *N. Engl. J. Med.*, 70:597, 1964.

Javid M.: Treatment of herniated lumbar disc syndrome with chymopapain. *JAMA* 243:2043, 1980.
[*A concise, current follow-up study of intradiscal therapy with chymopapain.*]

Jennett W.B.: A study of 25 cases of compression of the cauda equina by prolapsed intervertebral discs. *J. Neurol. Neurosurg. Psychiatry* 19:109, 1956.
[*An important review of the cauda equina syndrome in disc displacement.*]

Jones D.L., Moore T.: The types of neuropathic bladder dysfunction associated with prolapsed lumbar intervertebral discs. *Br. J. Urol.* 45:39, 1973.
[*An excellent description of early symptoms of lower motor neuron neurogenic bladder.*]

Joplin R.J.: The intervertebral disc: Embryology, anatomy, physiology and pathology. *Surg. Gynecol. Obstet.* 61:591, 1935.

Joshi P.N., Shankar V., Abraham K.I., et al.: Separation of chymopapain from papaya latex (Carica papaya) on amberlite IR-120 (Hb2 +). *J. Chromatogr.* 121:65, 1976.

Joyce C.R.B.: Consistent differences in individual reactions to drugs and dummies. *Br. J. Pharmacol.* 14:512, 1959.

Kanazawa H., Ishimitsu S., Skane M., et al.: Chymopapain: II. Photooxidation of histidine residues. *Chem. Pharm. Bull. (Tokyo)* 24(12):3088, 1976.

Kanazawa H., Ishimitsu S., Skane M., et al.: Chymopapain: I. Oxidation of tryptophan residues by *n*-bromosuccinimide. *Chem. Pharm. Bull. (Tokyo)* 24(10):2369, 1976.

Kaplan R.: Sensitivity reaction: Chymopapain vs radiographic dye, letter. *Anesthesiology* 47:399, 1977.

Kapsalis A.A., Stern I.J.: Detection of chymopapain immunoreactive protein (C1) in canine and human plasma by radioimmunoassay, in *Proceedings of the Fifth International Congress on Pharmacology.* 1972, p. 119.

Kapsalis A.A., Stern I.J., Bernstein I.: The fate of chymopapain injected for therapy in intervertebral disk disease. *J. Lab. Clin. Med.* 83:532, 1974.
[*An excellent basic science study on the fate of intradiscally injected chymopapain.*]

Katsura N., Davidson E.S.: Metabolism of connective tissue polysaccharides in vivo: IV. The sulphate group. *Biochem. Biophys. Acta* 121:135, 1966.

Katz A.M., Battit G.E., Wilkey B.R.: An anaphylactoid reaction to penicillin during anesthesia. *Anesthesiology* 32:84, 1970.

Keck C.: Discography, technique and interpretation. *Arch. Surg.* 80:580, 1960.

Keegan J.: Dermatome hypalgesia associated with herniation of intervertebral disk. *Arch. Neurol.* 50:67, 1943.

Keegan J.: Diagnosis of herniation of lumbar intervertebral disc by neurological signs. *JAMA* 126:868, 1944.

Keeney E., Weiss H., Mohr C.: The use of cortisone or ACTH during rapid desensitization of allergic patients. *J. Allergy* 26:141, 1955.

Kelly J., Patterson R.: Anaphylaxis: Course, mechanism and treatment. *JAMA* 227:1431, 1974.
[*A good review of anaphylaxis.*]

Kelly J., Patterson R., Lieberman P., et al.: Radiographic contrast media studies in high risk patients. *J. Allergy Clin. Immunol.* 62:181, 1978.
[*One of several studies demonstrating some protective effect of diphenhydramine and hydrocortisone against anaphylactic reaction.*]

Kelly M.: Physical changes in the prolapsed disc. *Lancet* 7046:584, 1968.

Kendall P.H., Jenkins J.M.: Exercises for backache: A double-blind controlled trial. *Physiotherapy* 54:154, 1968.
[*A frequently cited early attempt at a controlled prospective study on the treatment of backache.*]

Kern R.A.: Anaphylactic drug reactions: Their diagnosis, prevention and treatment. *JAMA* 179:19, 1962.

Key J.A.: Low back pain as seen in an orthopedic clinic. *Am. J. Med. Sci.* 168:526, 1924.

Key J.A., Ford L.T.: Experimental intervertebral disc lesions. *J. Bone Joint Surg.* 30-A:621, 1948.

Key J.A.: The intervertebral disk: Anatomy, physiology and pathology, in American Academy of Orthopedic Surgeons: *Instructional Course Lectures.* Ann Arbor, J.W. Edwards Co., 1954, No. 11, p. 101.

Key J.A.: Intervertebral disk lesions and low-back pain, in American Academy of Orthopedic Surgeons: *Instructional Course Lectures.* Ann Arbor, J.W. Edwards Co., 1954, No. 11, p. 99.

Keyes D.C., Compere E.L.: The normal and pathological physiology of the nucleus pulposus of the intervertebral disc: An anatomical, clinical and experimental study. *J. Bone Joint Surg.* 14:897, 1932.

Kime J., Fancher O.E., Calandra J.C.: *Industrial Bio-Test Laboratories, Inc. Report to Baxter Laboratories,* publication No. IBTA-3144. Morton Grove, Ill., April 1, 1966.

Kimmel J.R., Smith E.L.: Crystalline papain: I. Preparation, specificity, and activation. *J. Biol. Chem.* 207:515, 1954.

King A.S., Smith R.N.: A comparison of the anatomy of the intervertebral disk in dog and man. *Br. Vet. J.* 3:135, 1955.

King J.S., Lagger R.: Sciatica viewed as a referred pain syndrome. *Surg. Neurol.* 5:46, 1976.

Kitchell J.R., Glover R.P., Kyle R.H.: Bilateral internal mammary artery ligation for angina pectoris: Preliminary clinical considerations. *Am. J. Cardiol.* 1:46, 1958.

Knighton R.S.: Evaluation of the authenticity of the controlled double blind study of chymopapain. Letter to Baxter Travenol Laboratories, 1975.

Knutsson B.: Electromyographic studies on the diagnosis of lumbar disc herniations. *Acta Orthop. Scand.* 28:390, 1959.

Knutsson B.: How often do the neurological signs disappear after the operation of a herniated disc? *Acta Orthop. Scand.* 32:352, 1962.
[*Data from this study were used to compare surgery with chymopapain for the reversal of neurologic deficit.*]

Knutsson B., Wiberg G.: On surgically treated herniated intervertebral discs. *Acta Orthop. Scand.* 28:108, 1958.

Knutsson F.: The instability associated with disc degeneration in the lumbar spine. *Acta Radiol.* 25:593, 1944.
[*An early demonstration of mechanical insufficiency from disc degeneration.*]

Knutsson F.: Lumbar myelography with water-soluble contrast in cases of disc prolapse. *Acta Orthop. Scand.* 20:294, 1951.

Kokan P.: Chemonucleolysis. Read before a symposium on the application of proteolytic enzymes of carica papaya in broad clinical medicine, Moscow, 1978.

Kramer J.: Fluid exchange in the intervertebral disc and instillation therapy. Read before the Congress of the International Society for the Study of the Lumbar Spine, London, July 3, 1975.

Kraemer J., Keiko L.: Lumbar intradiscal instillation with aprotinin. *Spine* 7:73, 1982.
[*The clinical course in these patients gives some insight into the mechanism of pain production from disc displacement.*]

Kraemer J., Laturnus H.: Treatment of lumbar intervertebral disc lesions by intradiscal instillation of pressure-reducing substances. *Z. Orthop.* 113:1031, 1975.

Krempen J.F., Minnig D.E., Smith B.S.: Experimental studies on the effect of chymopapain on nerve root compression caused by intervertebral disk material. *Clin. Orthop.* 106:336, 1975.

Kuhns J.G.: Conservative treatment of sciatic pain in low back disability. *J. Bone Joint Surg.* 23:435, 1941.

Kunimitsu D.K.: *The Purification and Some Physical Chemical Traits of Crystalline Chymopapain B,* thesis. University of Hawaii, 1964.

Kunimitsu D.K., Yasumobu K.T.: Chymopapain: IV. The chromatographic fractionation of partially purified chymopapain and the characterization of crystalline chymopapain B. *Biochim. Biophys. Acta* 139:405, 1967.

Kunkel, M.: Chemonucleolysis. Read before the annual meeting of the Canadian Orthopedic Association, 1974.

Lasagna L., Masteller F., von Feisnger J.A., et al.: A study of the placebo response. *Am. J. Med.* 16:770, 1954.

Chymopapain and the intervertebral disc, editorial. *Lancet* 815–816, 1967.

Leavitt F., Garron D.C., Whisler W.W., et al.: Affective and sensory dimensions of back pain. *Pain* 4:273, 1978.

Leavitt F., Garron D.C., Whisler W.W., et al.: A comparison of patients treated by chymopapain and laminectomy for low back pain using a multidimensional pain scale. *Clin. Orthop.* 146:136, 1980.

Leavitt S.S., Johnston T.L., Beyer R.D.: The process of recovery: Patterns in industrial back injury. Part 2. Predicting outcomes from early case data. *Ind. Med. Surg.* 40:7, 1971.

Lehtonen A., Viljanto J., Karkkainen J.: The mucopolysaccharides of herniated human intervertebral discs and semilunar cartilages. *Acta Chir. Scand.* 133:303, 1967.

Levine B.: Immunologic mechanisms of penicillin allergy. *N. Engl. J. Med.* 275:1119, 1966.

Lewin T.: Osteoarthritis in lumbar synovial joints. *Acta Orthop. Scand. [Suppl.]* 43, 1964.

Lieberman P., Siegle R., Kaplan R., et al.: Chronic urticaria and intermittent anaphylaxis. *JAMA* 1232:495, 1976.

Linard de Guertechin D., Vincent A.: Intermediate term results of chemonucleolysis. *Acta Orthop. Belg.* 42:139, 1976.

Lind G.A.M.: *Autotraction: Treatment for Low Back Pain and Sciatica*, thesis. Linkopings University, Sweden, 1975.

Lindahl S., Brown M., Irstam L., et al.: Roentgenologic grading of disc degeneration by discography. Read by title before the International Society for the Study of the Lumbar Spine, Toronto, 1982.

Lindblom K.: Diagnostic puncture of intervertebral disks in sciatica. *Acta Orthop. Scand.* 1:231, 1948.

Lindblom K.: Technique and results in myelography and disc puncture. *Acta Radiol.* 34:321, 1950.

Lindblom K.: Technique and results of diagnostic disc puncture and injection (discography) in the lumbar region. *Acta Orthop. Scand.* 20:315, 1950.

Lindholm R., Salenius P.: Caudal, epidural administration of anesthetics and corticoids in the treatment of low back pain. *Acta Orthop. Scand.* 35:144, 1964.

Lindstrom A., Zachrisson M.: Physical therapy on low back pain and sciatica. *Scand. J. Rehabil. Med.* 2:37, 1970.

Lineweaver H., Schwinner S.: Some properties of crystalline papain: Stability toward heat, pH and urea; pH optimum with casein as substrate. *Enzyme* 10:81, 1941.

Loebl W.Y.: Measurements of spinal posture and range of spinal movement. *Ann. Phys. Med.* 9:103, 1967.

Loew F., Kivelitz R.: First results of a series of chemonucleolysis. *J. Neurol. Sci.* 17:77, 1973.

Logue V.: Chemonucleolysis. *J. Bone Joint Surg.* 49-B:401, 1967.

Love J.G.: Protrusion of the intervertebral disk (fibrocartilage) into the spinal canal. *Mayo Clin. Proc.* 11:529, 1936.

Love J.G.: Low back and sciatic pain. *Surg. Clin. North Am.* 19:943, 1939.

Love J.G.: Protruded intervertebral disks with a note regarding hypertrophy of ligamenta flava. *JAMA* 113:2029, 1939.

Love J.G.: Removal of protruded intervertebral disks without laminectomy. *Mayo Clin. Proc.* 14:800, 1939.

Love J.G., Rivers M.H.: Spinal cord tumors simulating protruded intervertebral disks. *JAMA* 179:878, 1962.
[*The differential diagnosis of disc displacement.*]

Love J.G., Walsh M.N.: Protruded intervertebral disks: A report of 100 cases in which operation was performed. *JAMA* 111:396, 1938.

Lowther D.A., Baxter E.: Isolation of a chondroitin sulphate protein complex from bovine intervertebral disks. *Nature* 2:595, 1966.

Luck J.B.: Psychosomatic problems in military orthopaedic surgery. *J. Bone Joint Surg.* 28:213, 1946.

Lundborg G.: Ischemic nerve injury: Experimental studies on intraneural microvascular pathophysiology and nerve function in a limb subjected to temporary circulatory arrest. *Scand. J Plast. Reconstr. Surg [Suppl.]* 6, 1970.

Lundborg G.: Structure and function of the intraneural microvessels as related to trauma, edema formation and nerve function. *J. Bone Joint Surg.* 57-A:938, 1975.
[*The classic study for the understanding of the pathophysiology of nerve injury.*]

Lundborg G., Brånemark P.-I.: Microvascular structure and function of peripheral nerves: Vital microscopic studies of the tibial nerve in rabbit. *Adv. Microcirc.* 1:66, 1968.

Lundskog J., Brånemark P.-I.: Microvascular proliferation produced by autologous grafts of nucleus pulposus. *Adv. Microcirc.* 3:115, 1970.

Lynn K.R.: An isolation of chymopapain. *J. Chromatogr.* 84:423, 1973.

Lyons H., Jones E., Quinn F.E., et al.: Protein-polysaccharide complexes of normal and herniated human intervertebral discs. *Proc. Soc. Exp. Biol. Med.* 115:610, 1964.

Lyons H., Jones E., Quinn F.E., et al.: Changes in the protein polysaccharide fractions of nucleus pulposus from human intervertebral disc with age and disc herniation. *J. Lab. Clin. Med.* 68:930, 1966.

Ma V.Y.N.: Experience with chymopapain injection into lumbar discs. *J. West. Pacific Orthop. Assoc.* 6:170, 1969.

MacLarin W., Aladjem F.: Allergy to chymotrypsin. *J. Allergy* 28:89, 1957.

MacNab I.: Negative disc exploration. *J. Bone Joint Surg.* 53-A:891, 1971.
[*Gives several reasons why chemonucleolysis might fail.*]

MacNab I.: Chemonucleolysis. *Clin. Neurosurg.* 20:183, 1973.

MacNab I.: Chemonucleolysis, in *Congress of Neurological Surgeons: Proceedings of the 22nd Annual Meeting, 1972.* Baltimore, Williams & Wilkins Co., 1973, p. 183.

MacNab I.: The surgery of lumbar disc degeneration, in Nyhus L.M. (ed.): *Surgery Annual*. New York, Appleton-Century-Crofts, 1976, vol. 8, p. 447.

MacNab I., McCullough J.A., Wiener D.S., et al.: Chemonucleolysis. *Can. J. Surgery* 14:280, 1971.
[*The first study clearly differentiating results of chemonucleolysis for pure disc displacement vs. spinal stenosis.*]

MacNab I., St. Louis E.L., Grabias S.L., et al.: Selective ascending lumbosacral venography in the assessment of lumbar disc herniation. *J. Bone Joint Surg.* 58-A:1093, 1976.
[*Technique is now obsolete because of CT imaging.*]

Magora A.: Investigation of the relation between low back pain and occupation: III. Physical requirements: sitting, standing and weight-lifting. *Ind. Med. Surg.* 41:5, 1972.

Magora A., Schwartz A.: Relation between the low back pain syndrome and x-ray findings. *Scand. J. Rehabil. Med.* 8:115, 1976.

Malawista I., Schubert M.: Chondromucoprotein: New extraction method and alkaline degradation. *J. Biol. Chem.* 230:535, 1958.

Mandl I.: Collagenase. *Science* 169:1234, 1970.

Mandl I., MacLennan J., Howes E.: Isolation and characterization of proteinase and collagenase from *Cl. Histolyticum. J. Clin. Invest.* 32:1312, 1953.
[*The original isolation of purified collagenase.*]

Mandl I., Zipper H., Ferguson L.T.: *Clostridium histolyticum* collagenase: Its purification and properties. *Arch. Biochem. Biophys.* 4:465, 1958.

Mankin H.J.: Herniated intervertebral disc: Chemo vs surgical vs expectant therapy. Read before the annual meeting of the American Association of Neurological Surgeons, Los Angeles, April, 1973.

Maroon J.C., Holst R.A., Osgood C.P.: Chymopapain in the treatment of ruptured lumbar discs: Preliminary experience in 48 patients. *J. Neurol. Neurosurg. Psychiatry* 39:508, 1976.

Marshall L.L.: Intradiscal enzyme for back pain, letter. *Med. J. Aust.* 2:616, 1973.

Marshall L.L., Trethewie E.R.: Chemical irritation of nerve roots in disc prolapse. *Lancet* 2:320, 1973.

Marshall W.J.S., Schorstein J.: Factors affecting the results of surgery for prolapsed lumbar intervertebral disc. *Scott. Med. J.* 13:38, 1968.

Martins A.N., Ramirez A., Johnston J., et al.: Double-blind evaluation of chemonucleolysis for herniated lumbar discs: Late results. *J. Neurosurg.* 49:816, 1978.
[*Patients with objective signs of disc displacement had better results with Discase than with CEI (placebo).*]

Maruta R., Swanson D.W., Swenson W.M.: Low back pain patients in a psychiatric population. *Mayo Clin. Proc.* 51:57, 1976.

Massaro T.A., Javid M.: Chemonucleolysis, letter. *J. Neurosurg.* 46:696, 1977.

Massie W. (ed.): *Symposium on Chemonucleolysis. Clin. Orthop.* 67:2, 1969.

Massie W.K., Stevens D.B.: A critical evaluation of discography. *J. Bone Joint Surg.* 49-A:1243, 1967.

Mathews M.B.: Isomeric chondroitin sulfates. *Nature* 181:421, 1958.

Mathews M.B.: The interaction of collagen and acid mucopolysaccharides: A model for connective tissue. *Biochem. J.* 96:710, 1965.

Mayfield F.H.: Complications of laminectomy. *Clin. Neurosurg.* 23:435, 1976.

McCluskey R.T., Thomas L.: Removal of cartilage matrix, in vivo, by papain: Identification of crystalline papain protease as cause of phenomenon. *J. Exp. Med.* 108:371, 1958.

McCulloch J.A.: Personal communication, August 1982.

McCulloch J.A.: Chemonucleolysis. *J. Bone Joint Surg.* 59-B:45, 1977.

McCulloch J.A.: Chemonucleolysis: Experience with 2,000 cases. *Clin. Orthop.* 146:128, 1980.
[*The largest clinical series of intradiscal therapy by one surgeon.*]

McCulloch J.A.: Chemonucleolysis for relief of sciatica due to a herniated intervertebral disc. *CMA J.* 124:879, 1981.

McCulloch J.A.: Chemonucleolysis, letter. *CMA J.* 126:119, 1982.

McCulloch J.A.: Computed tomography before and after chemonucleolysis, in Post M.J.D. (ed.): *Computer Tomography of the Spine.* Baltimore, Williams & Wilkins Co., 1983, chap. 25.

McCulloch J.A., Ferguson J.: Outpatient chemonucleolysis. *Spine* 6:606, 1981.
[*It can be done safely, according to this report and subsequent extensive experience by the senior author.*]

McCulloch J.A., Waddell G.: Lateral lumbar discography. *Br. J. Radiol.* 51:498, 1978.

McGill C.M.: Industrial back problems: A controlled program. *J. Occup. Med.* 10:174, 1968.

McKenzie Johnston R.: Notes on the use of papain in ear disease. *Edinburgh Med. J.* 35:621, 1890.

McKinley J.C., Hathaway S.R.: The identification and measurement of the psychoneuroses in medical practice: The Minnesota Multiphasic Personality Inventory. *JAMA* 122:161, 1943.

McLellon A.T., Lubrosky L., O'Brien C.P., et al.: Is treatment for substance abuse effective? *JAMA* 248:1423, 1982.
[*An important article for physicians treating patients in pain.*]

McNeill T., Huncke B., Pesch R.N.: Chemonucleolysis: Evaluation of effectiveness by electromyography. *Arch. Phys. Med. Rehabil.* 58:303, 1977.

McPherson K.: Statistics: The problem of examining accumulating data more than once. *N. Engl. J. Med.* 290:501, 1974.

Meyerding H.W.: Low backache and sciatic pain associated with spondylolisthesis and protruded intervertebral disc: Incidence, significance and treatment. *J. Bone Joint Surg.* 23:461, 1941.

Middleton G.S., Teacher J.H.: Injury of the spinal cord due to rupture of an intervertebral disc during muscular effort. *Glasgow Med. J.* 76:1, 1911.

Milward F.J., Grant J.L.A.: Changes in the intervertebral discs following lumbar puncture. *Lancet* 2:183, 1936.

Mineiro J.D.: *Coluna Vertebral Humana: Alguna Aspecta da sua Estruturae Vascularizacao,* thesis. University of Lisbon, 1965.

Mitchell P.E.G., Hendry N.G.C., Billewicz W.Z.: The chemical background of intervertebral disk prolapse. *J. Bone Joint Surg.* 43-B:141, 1961.
[*Classic description of the biochemical basis for disc displacement.*]

Mixter W.J.: Rupture of the lumbar intervertebral disk: An etiologic factor for so-called "sciatic" pain. *Ann. Surg.* 106:777, 1937

Moertel D.G., Taylor W.F., Roth A., et al.: Who responds to sugar pills? *Mayo Clin. Proc.* 51:96, 1976.

Mount H.T.R.: Hydrocortisone in the treatment of intervertebral disc protrusion. *Can. Med. Assoc. J.* 105:1279, 1971.

Murphy F.: Sources and patterns of pain in disc disease. *Clin. Neurosurg.* 15:343, 1968.

Nachemson A.: Some mechanical properties of the lumbar intervertebral disc. *Bull. Hosp. Joint Diseases* 23:130, 1962.

Nachemson A.: The influence of spinal movements on the lumbar intradiscal pressure and on the tensile stresses in the annulus fibrosa. *Acta Orthop. Scand.* 33:183, 1963.

Nachemson A.: The effect of forward leaning on lumbar intradiscal pressure. *Acta Orthop. Scand.* 34:314, 1965.

Nachemson A.: In vivo discometry in lumbar discs with irregular nucleograms. *Acta Orthop. Scand.* 36:418, 1965.

Nachemson A.: The load on lumbar disks in different positions of the body. *Clin. Orthop.* 45:107, 1966.

Nachemson A.: Oxphenylbutazon in surgery for herniated discs: A double blind trial. *Acta Orthop. Scand.* 37:267, 1966.

Nachemson A.: Intradiscal measurement of pH in patients with lumbar rhizopathies. *Acta Orthop. Scand.* 40:23, 1969.

Nachemson A.: Physiotherapy for low back patients. *Scand. J. Rehabil. Med.* 1:85, 1969.
[*One of many admonitions by this author to base treatment on the results of controlled studies.*]

Nachemson A.: Low back pain: Its etiology and treatment. *Clin. Med.* 78:18, 1971.

Nachemson A.: The lumbar spine, an orthopedic challenge. *Spine* 1:59, 1976.

Nachemson A., Ejeskar A., Herverts P., et al.: Chymopapain injection for disc hernia: Preliminary results of a controlled study. *Acta Orthop. Scand.* 48:216, 1977.

Nachemson A., Elfstrom G.: Intravital dynamic pressure measurements in lumbar discs. *Scand. J. Rehabil. Med.* 1:1, 1970.

Nachemson A., Morris J.M.: In vivo measurements of intradiscal pressure discometry: A method for the determination of pressure in the lower lumbar discs. *J. Bone Joint Surg.* 46-A:1077, 1964.

Nahum L.H.: Chemical removal of nucleus pulposus. *Conn. Med.* 28:507, 1964.

National Center for Health Statistics: *Hospital Discharge Survey,* Bethesda, 1968.

Natvig H.: Sociomedical aspects of low back pain causing prolonged sick-leave: A retrospective study. *Acta Sociomed. Scand.* 2:117, 1970.

Naylor A.: Changes in the human intervertebral disc with age. *Proc. R. Soc. Med.* 51:573, 1958.

Naylor A.: The biophysical and biochemical aspects of intervertebral disc herniation and degeneration. *Ann. R. Coll. Surg.* 31:91, 1962.

Naylor A.: The biochemical changes in the human intervertebral disc in degeneration and nuclear prolapse. *Orthop. Clin. North Am.* 2:343, 1971.

Naylor A., Earland C., Robinson J.: The effect of diagnostic radio-opaque fluids used in discography on chymopapain activity. *Spine,* to be published.
[*Reassurance of the lack of inhibition of the action of chymopapain on the disc by radio-contrast dyes used in discography.*]

Naylor A., Happey F., MacRae T.: The collagenous changes in the intervertebral disk with age and their effect on its elasticity: An x-ray crystallographic study. *Br. Med.* 2:570, 1954.

Nies A., Melman K.: Kinins and arthritis. *Bull. Rheum. Dis.* 19:512, 1968.

Nordby E.J.: Forum: Chymopapain. *Spine* 2:231, 1977.

Nordby E.J.: A method for lateral discography and chemonucleolysis. *Spectator Letter, Chymopapain Workshop,* Jan. 20, 1979.

Nordby E.J.: Personal communication, August 1982.

Nordby E.J., Brown M.D.: Present status of chymopapain and chemonucleolysis. *Clin. Orthop.* 129:79, 1977.
[*Historical review and correlation of clinical and research data on chymopapain.*]

Nordby E.J., Lucas G.L.: A comparative analysis of lumbar disc disease treated by laminectomy or chemonucleolysis. *Clin. Orthop.* 90:119, 1973.

Nulsen F.: Herniated intervertebral disc: Chemo vs surgical vs expectant therapy. Read before the annual meeting of the American Association of Neurological Surgeons, Los Angeles, 1973.

O'Connell J.E.A.: Protrusions of lumbar intervertebral discs: A clinical review based on 5,000 cases treated by excision of the protrusion. *J. Bone Joint Surg.* 33-B:8, 1951.
[*An important clinical follow-up study on the surgical treatment of disc displacement.*]

O'Dell C.W., Coel M.N., Ignelzi R.J.: Ascending lumbar venography in lumbar-disc disease. *J. Bone Joint Surg.* 59-A:159, 1977.

Onofrio B.M.: Injection of chymopapain into intervertebral discs: Preliminary report on 72 patients with symptoms of disc disease. *J. Neurosurg.* 42:384, 1975.
[*Very well-documented clinical trial of chymopapain for intradiscal therapy.*]

Orange R., Donsky G.: Anaphylaxis, in Middleton E., Reed C., Ellis E. (eds.): *Allergy Principles and Practice.* St. Louis, C.V. Mosby Co., vol. 2, 1978, p. 563.

Ortho-Tex Laboratories: *Chemolase Protocol.* San Antonio, Ortho-Tex Laboratories, June 1982.

Ottolenghi C.E.: Aspiration biopsy of the spine. *J. Bone Joint Surg.* 51-A:1531, 1969.

Parkinson D.: Treatment with chymopapain, letter. *J. Neurosurg.* 39:794, 1973.

Parkinson D., Shields C.: Treatment of protruded lumbar intervertebral discs with chymopapain (Discase). *J. Neurosurg.* 39:203, 1973.

Patrick B.S.: Lumbar discography: A five year study. *Surg. Neurol.* 1:267, 1973.

Paulson S., Sylven B., Hirsch C., et al.: Biophysical and physiological investigations on cartilage and other mesenchymal tissues: III. The diffusion rate of various substances in normal bovine nucleus pulposus. *Biochim. Biophys. Acta* 7:207, 1951.

Pearce J., Moll J.M. II: Conservative treatment and natural history of acute lumbar disc lesions. *J. Neurol. Neurosurg. Psychiatry* 30:13, 1967.
[*The first article that clearly documented the high rate of spontanous remission of symptoms of disc displacement.*]

Pedersen H.E., Blunck C.G.J., Gardner E.: The anatomy of the lumbosacral posterior rami and meningeal branches of spinal nerves (sinu-vertebral nerves). *J. Bone Joint Surg.* 38-A:377, 1956.

Peto R., Pike M., Armitage P., et al.: Design and analysis of randomized clinical trials requiring prolonged observation of each patient. *Br. J. Cancer* 34:585, 1976.

Petter C.K.: Methods of measuring the pressure of the intervertebral disc. *J. Bone Joint Surg.* 15:365, 1933.

Pheasant H.: Backache: Its nature, incidence and cost. *Western J. Med.* 126:330, 1977.
[*Analysis of the medical cost associated with backache.*]

Philbin D.M., Moss J., Akins C.W., et al.: The use of H_1- and H_2- histamine antagonists with morphine anesthesia: A double-blind study. *Anesthesiology* 55:292, 1981.
[*If results are applicable in control of severity of anaphylaxis, this will be an important reference for those using chymopapain.*]

Phillipa E.L.: Some psychological characteristics associated with orthopaedic complaints. *Curr. Pract. Orthop. Surg.* 2:165, 1964.

Phillips O., Ebner H., Nelson A., et al.: Neurologic complications following spinal anesthesia with lidocaine. *Anesthesiology* 30:284, 1969.

Pilling L.F., Brannick T.L., Swenson W.M.: Psychological characteristics of psychiatric patients having pain as a presenting symptom. *Can. Med. Assoc. J.* 97:387, 1967.

Popovic J., Tabor L., Cerk M.: Nucleolysis by papain in intervertebral disc herniation. *Rheumatizam (Zagreb)* 22:16, 1975.

Post J.D., Brown M.D., Gargano F.P.: The technique and interpretation of lumbar myelograms. *Spine* 2:214, 1977.

Post M.J.D.: CT update: The impact of time, metrizamide, and high resolution on the diagnosis of spinal pathology, in Post M.J.D. (ed.): *Radiographic Evaluation of the Spine: Current Advances with Emphasis on Computer Tomography.* New York, Masson Publishers, 1980, pp. 259–294.
[*The second edition will be published in 1983.*]

Potter J.L., McCluskey R.T., Weissman G., et al.: The effect of papain on cartilage in vivo: Factors influencing the distribution of papain protease following intravenous injection. *Ann. NY Acad. Sci.* 86:929, 1960.

Potter J.L., McCluskey R.T., Weissman G., et al.: Removal of cartilage matrix by papain: Factors affecting distribution of crystalline papain in vivo. *J. Exp. Med.* 112:1173, 1960.

Prieur D.J., Young D.M., Davis R.D.: Procedures for preclinical toxicologic evaluation of cancer chemotherapeutic agents: Part 3. Protocols of the Laboratory of Toxicology. *Cancer Chemother. Rep.* 4:10, 1973.

Putti V.: The Lady Jones Lecture: Pathogenesis of sciatic pain. *Lancet* 2:53, 1927.

Quinnel R., Stockdale H.: An investigation of artifacts in lumbar discography. *Br. J. Radiol.* 53:831, 1980.
[*An important observation in interpreting discograms.*]

Raaf J.: Some observations regarding 905 patients operated on for protruded intervertebral disc. *Am. J. Surg.* 9:388, 1959.

Rabinovich R.: *Diseases of the Intervertebral Disc and its Surrounding Tissues.* Springfield, Ill., Charles C Thomas, Publisher, 1961, p. 152.

Rajagopalan R., Tindal S., MacNab I.: Anaphylactic reactions to chymopapain during general anesthesia: A case report. *Anesth. Analg.* 53:191, 1974.

Ramani P.: Variations in size of the bony lumbar canal in patients with prolapse of lumbar intervertebral discs. *Clin. Radiol.* 27:301, 1976.

Ramsey R.H.: Conservative treatment of intervertebral disk lesions, in American Academy of Orthopedic Surgeons: *Instructional Course Lectures.* Ann Arbor, J.W. Edwards Co., 1954, No. 11, p. 118.

Ransford A.D., Carrins D., Mooney V.: The pain drawing as an aid to the psychologic evaluation of patients with low back pain. *Spine* 1:127, 1976.
[*A helpful diagnostic tool.*]

Ransford A.D., Harries B.J.: Localized arachnoiditis complicating lumbar lesions. *J. Bone Joint Surg.* 54-B:656, 1972.

Reynolds F.C.: Report on a double-blind study to the American Academy of Orthopaedic Surgeons, letter. Nov. 7, 1975.

Reynolds F.C., McGinnis A.E., Morgan H.C.: Surgery in the treatment of low back pain and sciatica. *J. Bone Joint Surg.* 41:223, 1959.

Ripley H.S.: The physiological basis of pain, in Bonica J.J.: *The Management of Pain.* Philadelphia, Lea & Febiger, 1953, p. 143.

Rissanen P.M.: The surgical anatomy and pathology of the supraspinous and interspinous ligaments of the lumbar spine with special reference to ligament ruptures. *Acta Orthop. Scand. [Suppl.]* 46, 1960.

Roland M., Morris R.: A study of the natural history of back pain: I. Development of a reliable and sensitive measure of disability in low back pain. *Spine,* to be published.
[*This will be a better method of determining the outcome of treatment.*]

Roland M., Morris R.: A study of the natural history of back pain: II. Development of guidelines for trials of treatment in primary care. *Spine,* to be published.

Roofe P.G.: Innervation of annulus fibrosus and posterior longitudinal ligament. *Arch. Neurol.* 44:100, 1940.

Rose K.: Anaphylactic reaction to aqueous chymotrypsin injection. *JAMA* 173:796, 1960.

Rosen H.: Letter. *Can. Med. Assoc. J.* 125:2445, 1981.

Rosen H.J.: Lumbar intervertebral disc surgery: Review of 300 cases. *Can. Med. Assoc. J.* 101:317, 1969.

Rosenberg L., Schubert M.: The proteinpolysaccharides of bovine nucleus pulposus. *J. Biol. Chem.* 242:4691, 1967.

Roslund J.: *Indications for Lumbar Disc Surgery,* thesis. Stockholm, Tryckeri Balder AB, 1974.

Russell A.S.: Chymopapain chemonucleolysis in lumbar disk disease. *JAMA* 233:1164, 1975.

Rydevik B., Brånemark P.-I., Nordberg C., et al.: Effects of chymopapain on nerve tissue. *Spine* 1:137, 1976.
[*An important study for an understanding of the pathophysiologic basis for the neurotoxicity of chymopapain.*]

Rydevik B., Brown M.D., Ehira T.: Does nucleus pulposus have an irritating effect on nerve tissue? Read before the International Society for the Study of the Lumbar Spine, Toronto, June 1982.

Rydevik B., Brown M.D., Ehira T., et al.: Effects of collagenase on nerve tissue. Read before the International Society for the Study of the Lumbar Spine, Toronto, June 1982.

Sabiston D.C. Jr., Blalock A.: Experimental ligation of internal mammary artery and its effect on coronary occlusion. *Surgery* 43:906, 1958.

Salenius P., Laurent L.: Results of operative treatment of lumbar disc herniation. *Acta Orthop. Scand.* 48:630, 1977.

Sampson P.: Chymopapain: A case study in federal drug regulation. *JAMA* 240:195, 1978.

Sandoz I., Hodges C.V.: Uretheral injury incident to lumbar disc operation. *J. Urology* 93:687, 1965.

Saunders E.C.: Treatment of the canine intervertebral disc syndrome with chymopapain. *J. Am. Vet. Med. Assoc.* 145:893, 1964.

Saunders J.B., Inman V.T.: Pathology of the intervertebral disk. *Arch. Surg.* 40:389, 1940.

Schatzker J., Pennal G.F.: Spinal stenosis, a cause of cauda equina compression. *J. Bone Joint Surg.* 50-B:606, 1968.

Schgal A.D., Gardner W.J.: Corticosteriods administered intradurally for relief of sciatica. *Cleve. Clin. Qt.* 27:198, 1960.

Schneider R.C.: Position statement on chymopapain from the American Association of Neurological Surgeons. *J. Neurosurg.* 43:373, 1975.

Schoedinger G.R. 3rd, Ford L.T. Jr.: The use of chymopapain in ruptured lumbar discs. *South. Med. J.* 64:333, 1971.

Schöning B., Lorenz W., Doenicke A.: Prophylaxis of anaphylactoid reactions to a polypeptidal plasma substitute by H_1- and H_2-receptor antagonists: Synopsis of three randomized controlled trials. *Klin. Wochenschr.* 60:1048, 1982.
[*May have important application to the prophylaxis of the disastrous results of severe systemic allergic reactions.*]

Schubert M.: Intercellular macromolecules containing polysaccharides. *Biophys. J.* 4:119, 1964.

Schubert M., Hamerman D.: Metachromasia: Chemical theory and histochemical use. *J. Histochem Cytochem.* 4:159, 1956.

Schultz H., Fleming J.F.R., Vanderlinden R.G.: Results of chemonucleolysis in disc patients. Read before the Congress of Neurological Sciences, Vancouver, 1978.

Schwetschenau P.R., Ramirez A., Johnston J., et al.: Double-blind evaluations of intradiscal chymopapain for herniated lumbar discs: Early results. *J. Neurosurg.* 45:622, 1976.
[*One of three publications on the results of the original double-blind study of chymopapain.*]

Scoville W.B.: Letter to members of the American Association of Neurological Surgeons, 1974.

Scoville W.B., Corkill G.: Lumbar disc surgery: Technique of radical removal and early mobilization. *J. Neurosurg.* 39:265, 1973.

Scoville W.B., Silver D.: Results of Scoville and Silver's questionnaire on chymopapain, letter. *J. Neurosurg.* 42:487, 1975.

Seifter S., Gallop P.M., Klein L., et al.: Studies on collagen: II. Properties of purified collagenase and its inhibition. *J. Biol. Chem.* 234:285, 1959.

Seigel S., Heimlich E.: Anaphylaxis. *Pediatr. Clin. North Am.* 9:29, 1962.

Sewing K.-Fr.: Effects and side effects of H_1- and H_2-receptor antagonists in clinical situations. *Klin. Wochenschr.* 60:1046, 1982.

Shaffer J.W., Nussbaum K., Little J.M.: M.M.P.I. profiles of disability insurance claimants. *Am. J. Psychiatry* 129:403, 1972.

Shannon N., Paul E.: L4-5 and L5-S1 disc protrusions: Analysis of 323 cases operated on over 12 years. *J. Neurol. Neurosurg. Psychiatry* 42:804, 1979.

Shanta T.R., Bourne G.H.: The perineurial epithelium: A new concept, in Bourne G.H. (ed.): *The Structure and Function of Nervous Tissue.* New York, Academic Press, vol. 1, 1968, p. 379.

Shealy C.N.: Dangers of spinal injections without proper diagnosis. *JAMA* 197:156, 1966.

Shealy C.N.: Tissue reactions to chymopapain in cats. *J. Neurosurg.* 26:327, 1967.

Shealy C.N.: Transcript of proceedings, Subcommittee on Health of the Committee on Labor and Public Welfare, Subcommittee on Administrative Practice and Procedures of the Committee on Judiciary. Investigation into the Food and Drug Administration, portion relating to Discase. Washington, D.C., 1974, p. 103.

Shields C.B.: Chemonucleolysis. *J. Ky. Med. Assoc.* 3:259, 1975.

Shinners B.M., Hamby W.B.: Protruded lumbar intervertebral discs: Results following surgical and non-surgical therapy. *J. Neurosurg.* 6:450, 1949.

Simmons E.H., Segil C.M.: An evaluation of discography in the localization of symptomatic levels in discogenic disease of the spine. *Clin. Orthop.* 108:57, 1975.

Simmons J., Reitman J.: *The Status of Chemonucleolysis in the State of Texas and Anesthesia Management for Chemonucleolysis.* Ortho-Texas Laboratories, San Antonio, Texas, March 1, 1980.

Skalpe I.O., Torbergsen T., Amundsen P., et al.: Lumbar myelography with metrizamide. *Acta Radiol. [Suppl.] (Stockh.)* 335:367, 1973.

Slater R., Wild W., Hyman W.: Chymopapain series compared with laminotomy and/or laminectomy. Read before the Western Neurosurgical Society, Santa Barbara, Oct. 27–30, 1974.

Slepian A.: Lumbar disk surgery: Long follow-up results from three neurosurgeons. *NY State J. Med.* 66:1063, 1966.

Smare D.L., Happey F., Naylor A.: Physical changes in the prolapsed disc. *Lancet* 7038:157, 1968.

Smith E.L., Kimmel J.R., Brown D.M., et al.: Papaya lysozyme. *J. Biol. Chem.* 215:65, 1955.

Smith L.: Enzyme dissolution of nucleus pulposus in humans. *JAMA* 18:137, 1964.
[*First report of the clinical application of chymopapain for intradiscal therapy for symptomatic disc displacement.*]

Smith L.: Chemonucleolysis. *Clin. Orthop.* 67:72, 1969.
[*The term "chemonucleolysis" coined.*]

Smith L.: Chemonucleolysis, abstracted. *J. Bone Joint Surg.* 54-A:1975, 1972.

Smith L.: The ruptured lumbar disc. Read before the annual meeting of the American Association of Orthopedic Surgeons, Washington, Feb. 1972.

Smith L.: Failures with chemonucleolysis. *Orthop. Clin. North Am.* 1:255, 1975.
[*Excellent analysis of the reasons why chymopapain fails to relieve symptoms.*]

Smith L., Brown J.E.: Experiences with enzyme dissolution of the nucleus pulposus. Read before the 4th Combined Orthopedic Meeting, Vancover, British Columbia, June 16, 1964.

Smith L., Brown J.E.: Treatment of lumbar intervertebral disc lesions by direct injection of chymopapain. *J. Bone Joint Surg.* 49-B:502, 1967.
[*The classic original follow-up report on patients in whom chymopapain was used for symptomatic disc displacement.*]

Smith L., Garvin P.J., Jennings R.B.: Enzyme dissolution of the nucleus pulposus. *Nature* 198:1311, 1963.
[*Chymopapain is advocated for intradiscal therapy.*]

Smith L., Stern T.J.: Remarks before the Workshop on Cartilage Degradation and Repair, Washington, D.C., Nov. 2–5, 1966.

Smyth M.J., Wright W.W.: Sciatica and the intervertebral disc. *J. Bone Joint Surg.* 40-A:1401, 1958.

Sniper W.: The estimation and comparison of histamine release by muscle relaxants in man. *Br. J. Anaesth.* 24:232, 1952.

Snoek W., Wever H., Jorgensen B.: Double blind evaluation of extradural methyl prednisolone for herniated lumbar discs. *Acta Orthop. Scand.* 48:635, 1977.

Soderberg L.: Prognosis in conservatively treated sciatica. *Acta Orthop. Scand.* [*Suppl.*] 21:1, 1956.
[*Describes the natural history of symptoms of disc displacement.*]

Sorbie C.: Chemonucleolysis in the treatment of lumbar disc protrusion. *CMA J.* 124:840, 1981.

Soule S.D.: Proteolytic enzymes. *Mo. Med.* 64:918, 1967.

Spackmann D.H., Stein W.H., Moore S.: Automatic recording apparatus for use in the chromatography of amino acids. *Anal. Chem.* 30:1190, 1958.

Spangfort E.V.: The lumbar disc herniation: A computer-aided analysis of 2,504 operations. *Acta Orthop. Scand* [*Suppl.*] 142:71, 1972.
[*A large clinical study on the operative treatment for disc displacement.*]

Spengler D.M., Freeman C.W.: Patient selection for lumbar discectomy. *Spine* 4:129, 1979.
[*Guide to patient selection for invasive treatment of disc displacement.*]

Spicer S.S., Bryant J.H.: Cartilage changes in papain-treated rabbits. *Am. J. Pathol.* 33:1237, 1957.

Staffeldt E.S.: Conservative treatment of the sciatica syndrome. *Ugeskr. Laeger* 122:239, 1960.

Steindler A., Luck J.V.: Differential diagnosis of pain low in the back: Allocation of the source of pain by procaine hydrochloride method. *JAMA* 110:106, 1938.

Steinmetz J.: Dr. Lyman Smith tangles with the FDA over his papaya enzyme to treat bad backs. *People* 5:58, 1976.

Stern E.W., Coulson W.F.: Effects of collagenase upon the intervertebral disc in monkeys. *J. Neurosurg.* 44:32, 1976.

Stern I.J.: Biochemistry of chymopapain. *Clin. Orthop.* 6:42, 1969.

Stern I.J., Cosmas F., Smith L.: Urinary polyuronide excretion in man after enzymic dissolution of the chondromucous protein of the intervertebral disc or surgical stress. *Clin. Chim. Acta* 21:181, 1968.

Stern I.J., Smith L.: Dissolution by chymopapain in vitro of tissue from normal or prolapsed intervertebral disks. *Clin. Orthop.* 50:269, 1967.
[*Some indications of the rapidity of the enzymatic action of chymopapain on proteoglycans of the disc.*]

Stern W.E.: Studies on the in vivo effects of collagenase on the primate intervertebral disc. Read before the annual meeting of the Society of Neurological Surgeons, Los Angeles, April 1974.

Sternback R.A., Murphy R.W., Akeson W.H., et al.: Chronic low back pain, the "low back loser." *Postgrad. Med.* 53:135, 1973.

Stevens R., Dondi P., Muir H.: Proteoglycans of the intervertebral disc. *Biochem. J.* 179:573, 1979.

Stewart W.J.: Lateral discograms and chemonucleolysis in the treatment of ruptured or deteriorated lumbar discs. *Clin. Orthop.* 67:88, 1969.

Stockwell R.A., Barnett C.H.: Changes in permeability of articular cartilage with age. *Nature* 201:835, 1964.

Sullivan M.: Chemonucleolysis. *Proc. R. Soc. Med.* 68:479, 1975.

Sussman B., Bromley J., Gomez J.: Injection of collagenase in the treatment of herniated lumbar disk. *JAMA* 245:730, 1981.
[*The first report of a clinical follow-up series in which collagenase was used for intradiscal therapy for proven disc displacement.*]

Sussman B., Verly G.: *Collagenase and Chymopapain: A Study of Toxicity.* Washington, D.C., Howard University College of Medicine, 1975. [*Presented at the American Association of Surgeons*]

Sussman B.J.: Intervertebral discolysis with collagenase. *J. Natl. Med. Assoc.* 60:184, 1968. [*The first report on the use of collagenase to dissolve discs.*]

Sussman B.J.: Experimental intervertebral discolysis: A critique of collagenase and chymopapain applications. *Clin. Orthop.* 80:181, 1971.

Sussman B.J.: Treatment with chymopapain, letter. *J. Neurosurg.* 39:793, 1973.

Sussman B.J.: The question of experimental trial of chymopapain. *Orthop. Audio. Synopsis* 6:3, 1974.

Sussman B.J.: Chymopapain chemonucleolysis in lumbar disk disease, letter. *JAMA* 234:271, 1975.

Sussman B.J.: Inadequacies and hazards of chymopapain injections as treatment for intervertebral disc disease. *J. Neurosurg.* 42:389, 1975.

Sussman B.J., Mann M.: Experimental intervertebral discolysis with collagenase. *J. Neurosurg.* 31:628, 1969.

Sussman B.J., Mann M.: Experimental intervertebral discolysis with collagenase; in Mandl J. (ed.): *Collagenase.* New York, Gordon and Breach, 1972, p. 101.

Swanson D., Swenson W., Maruta K., et al.: Program for managing chronic pain: I. Program description and characteristics of patients. *Mayo Clin. Proc.* 51:401, 1976.

Sylven B.: On the biology of nucleus pulposus. *Acta Orthop. Scand.* 20:275, 1950.

Sylvest J.: Treatment of disc prolapse by enzymatic breakdown of the nucleus pulposus. *Ugeskr. Laeger* 137:504, 1975.

Taylor T.K.F., Akeson W.H.: Intervertebral disc prolapse: A review of morphologic and biochemical knowledge concerning the nature of the prolapse. *Clin. Orthop.* 76:54, 1971.

Taylor T.K.F., Little K.: Intracellular matrix of the intervertebral disk in aging and in prolapse. *Nature* 208:384, 1965.

Thomas L.: Reversible collapse of rabbits' ears after intravenous papain and prevention of recovery by cortisone. *J. Exp. Med.* 104:245, 1956. [*The first experimental observation of the effects of papaya enzymes on the cartilage matrix.*]

Tibbetts J., Javid M.: Chymopapain in the management of protruded lumbar disc syndrome. Read before the annual meeting of the American Association of Neurological Surgeons, St. Louis, April 1974.

The great papaya fracas: Does the fruit extract really help back pain? *Time Magazine,* Feb. 27, 1978, p. 51.

Toole B.P., Lowther D.A.: Precipitation of collagen fibrils in vitro by protein polysaccharides. *Biochem. Res. Commun.* 29:515, 1967.

Torgerson W.R., Dotter W.E.: Comparative roentgenographic study of the asymptomatic and symptomatic lumbar spine. *J. Bone Joint Surg.* 58:850, 1976.

Toumey J.W., Poppen J.L., Hurley M.T.: Cauda equina tumors as a cause of low-back syndrome. *J. Bone Joint Surg.* 32-A:249, 1950.

Travenol Laboratories: IND 1004, 1973.

Travenol Research Summary, Discase 2S120:2, 1970.

Travenol Research Summary, Discase 2S120:3, 1970.

Travenol Research Summary, Discase 2S120:4 & 5, 1970.

Travenol Laboratories: *Discase: Research Summary.* Morton Grove, Ill., Travenol Laboratories, August 1970.

Travenol Laboratories: *Discase: Patient Attitude and Perception Study: Report by Rabin Research Company.* Morton Grove, Ill., Travenol Laboratories, June 1975.

Travenol Laboratories: Statistical analysis and tabulation of data resulting from discase double-blind trial. Memorandum, July 28, 1975.

Travenol Laboratories: *Research Summary on Cysteine-Edetate-Iothalamate (CEI) Injection and Chymopapain Injection.* Morton Grove, Ill., Travenol Laboratories, December 1978.

Travenol Laboratories: *Discase: Scientific Review.* Morton Grove, Ill., Travenol Laboratories, April 1979.

Travenol Laboratories: *Section III: The Clinical Summary of New Drug Application to the FDA—Safety and Efficacy.* Deerfield, Ill., Travenol Laboratories, August 1981.

Travenol Laboratories: *Chymopapain (Discase) and Cysteine, Edetate, Iothalamate (CEI Injection) Double Blind FDA-Travenol Laboratories Study.* Morton Grove, Ill., Travenol Laboratories, Protocol, February 1982.

Tsaltas T.T.F.: Papain-induced changes in rabbit cartilage. *J. Exp. Med.* 108:30, 1958.

Two investigators lose right to use chymopapain. *JAMA* 229:247, 1974.

U.S. Food and Drug Administration: Section 505 (i) of Federal Food, Drug and Cosmetic Act and Section 312 of title 21 of the Code of Federal Regulation. Washington, D.C., FDA,

Velasquez J., Gold M.: Anaphylactic reaction to cephalothin during anesthesia. *Anesthesiology* 43:476, 1975.

Verbiest H.: A radicular syndrome from developmental narrowing of the lumbar vertebral canal. *J. Bone Joint Surg.* 36:230, 1954. Vindication for a disk tenderizer: *Med. World News* 15:14, 1974.

Waddell G., Kummel E.G., Lotto W.N., et al.: Failed lumbar disc surgery and repeat surgery following industrial injuries. *J. Bone Joint Surg.* 61-A:201, 1979.

Waddell G., McCulloch J., Kummel E., et al.: Nonorganic physical signs in low back pain. *Spine* 5:117, 1980.
[*The confusing physical findings in patients with psychogenic regional pain syndrome.*]

Walter A.: Emotion and low back pain. *Applied Therapy* 8:868, 1966.

Walton R.P.: Behavior of papain in the peritoneal cavity. *J. Pharmacol. Exp. Ther.* 43:387, 1931.

Watts C.: Chemonucleolysis: An appeal for objectivity, letter. *J. Neurosurg.* 42:488, 1975.

Watts C.: Complications of chemonucleolysis for lumbar disc disease. *Neurosurgery* 1:2, 1977.
[*A complete documentation of the type and incidence of complications following the first 13,7000 chymopapain injections.*]

Watts C., Hutchinson G., Clark W.K.: Chemonucleolysis: A clinical correlation study. Read before the annual meeting of the American Association of Neurological Surgeons, St. Louis, April 1974.

Watts C., Hutchison G., Stern J., et al.: Comparison of intervertebral disc disease treatment by chymopapain injection and open surgery. *J. Neurosurg.* 42:397, 1975.

Watts C., Knighton R., Roulhac G.: Chymopapain treatment of intervertebral disc disease. *J. Neurosurg.* 42:374, 1975.

Watts C., Williams O.B., Goldstein G.: Sensitivity reactions to intradiscal injection of chymopapain during general anesthesia. *Anesthesiology* 44:437, 1976.

Weber H.: An evaluation of conservative and surgical treatment of lumbar disc protrusion. *J. Oslo City Hosp.* 20:810, 1970.

Weber H.: Traction therapy in sciatica due to disc prolapse. *J. Oslo City Hosp.* 23:167, 1973.

Weber H.: The effect of delayed disc surgery on muscular paresis. *Acta Orthop. Scand.* 46:631, 1975.

Weber H.: Lumbar disc herniation: A prospective study of prognostic factors including a controlled trial. *J. Oslo City Hosp.* 28:33, 1978.

Weber H.: Lumbar disc herniation: A controlled prospective study with 10 years' observation. *Spine,* to be published.
[*Ten-year follow-up prospective controlled study of operative vs. nonoperative treatment of proved disc displacement.*]

Weiner D.S., MacNab I.: Use of chymopapain in degenerative disc disease: Preliminary report. *Can. Med. Assoc. J.* 102:1252, 1970.

Wengler R.A.: Chemonucleolysis. *Minn. Med.* 56:579, 1973.

Werb Z., Burleigh M.C., Barrett A.J., et al.: The interaction of α_2-macroglobulin with proteinases. *Biochem. J.* 139:359, 1974.

Westerborn O.: The effect of papain on epiphyseal cartilage: A morphological and biochemical study. *Acta Chir. Scand. [Suppl.]* 270, 1961.

Westerman G., Corman A., Stelos P., et al.: Adverse reactions to penicillin. *JAMA* 198:173, 1966.

Westrin C.G.: Low back sick-listing: A nosological and medical insurance investigation. *J. Scand. Soc. Med. [Suppl.]* 7, 1973.

Whitman Armitage: Observations upon an anatomic variation of the lumbosacral joint: Its diagnosis and treatment. *J. Bone Joint Surg.* 6:808, 1924.

Wiberg G.: Back pain in relation to the nerve supply of the intervertebral disc. *Acta Orthop. Scand.* 19:211, 1949.

Widdowson W.L.: Effects of chymopapain in the intervertebral disk of the dog. *J. Am. Vet. Med. Assoc.* 150:608, 1967.

Widell E.H., Wiltse L.L., Bateman J.G., et al: Experiences with chymopapain chemonucleolysis with analysis of suboptimal results. Read before the annual meeting of the Western Orthopedic Association, Las Vegas, Feb. 1973.

Wiesel S., Bernini P., Rothman R., et al.: Effectiveness of epidural steriods in the treatment of sciatica: A double-blind clinical trial. Read before the International Society for the Study of the Lumbar Spine, Toronto, 1982.

Wiesel S.W., Rothman R.H.: Acute low back pain: An objective analysis of conservative therapy. *Clin. Orthop.* 143:290, 1979.

Wilfling F.J., Klonoff H., Kokan P.: Psychological, demographic and orthopaedic factors associated with prediction of outcome of spinal fusion. *Clin. Orthop.* 90:153, 1973.

Willey J.J., MacNab I., Wortzman G.: Lumbar discography and its clinical application. *Can. J. Surg.* 11:280, 1968.

Williams R.: Microlumbar discectomy: A conservative surgical approach to the virgin herniated lumbar disc. *Spine* 3:175, 1978.

Wiltse L.: Chymopapain chemonucleolysis: Indications and results. Symposium or chymopapain chemonucleolysis, Las Vegas, February 1973.

Wiltse L.: Letter to Fred C. Reynolds, M.D., Aug. 5, 1973.

Wiltse L.L.: Chymopapain chemonucleolysis in lumbar disk disease. *JAMA* 233:1164, 1975.

Wiltse L.L.: Chymopapain chemonucleolysis in lumbar disc disease, letter. *JAMA* 234:272, 1975.

Wiltse L.L.: Lumbar disc disease: Laminectomy vs chymopapain chemonucleolysis, letter. *JAMA* 234:703, 1975.

Wiltse L.L.: Psychological testing in predicting the success of low back surgery. *Orthop. Clin. North Am.* 6:317, 1975.

Wiltse L.L.: Chemonucleolysis in ideal candidates for laminectomy. *The Spectator,* June 30, 1978.

Wiltse L.L.: Chemonucleolysis in ideal candidates for laminectomy. Personal communication, July 19, 1978.

Wiltse L.L.: Chemonucleolysis in ideal candidates for laminectomy, letter. *The Spectator,* June 30, 1979.

Wiltse L.L.: Chemonucleolysis, MicKibbin B. (ed.): *Yearbook.* London, Churchill Livingston, to be published.

Wiltse L., Bilderback R.: Comparison of 100 primary laminectomies with 100 primary chemonucleolysis, special emphasis upon pain mechanism. Read before the annual meeting of the Western Orthopedic Association, Los Angeles, October 1971.

Wiltse L.L., Rocchio P.D.: Predicting success of low back surgery using psychological tests. Read before the annual meeting of the American Orthopedic Association, Hot Springs, Va., June 26, 1973.

Wiltse L.L., Rocchio P.D.: Preoperative psychological tests as predictors of success of chemonucleolysis in the treatment of the low back syndrome. *J. Bone Joint Surg.* 57-A:478, 1975.
[*A controlled study of treatment outcome in patients with one to five objective findings and normal or abnormal psychometrics.*]

Wiltse L.L., Widell E.H., Hansen A.Y.: Chymopapain chemonucleolysis in lumbar disc disease. *JAMA* 231:474, 1975.
[*A classic follow-up study on the results in patients who had received intradiscal chymopapain.*]

Wiltse L.L., Widell E.H., Yuan M.A.: Chymopapain chemonucleolysis failures. *Clin. Orthop.* 126:121, 1977.

Wiltse L.L., Wilson R.: Studies of the effect of diatrizoate sodium and meglumine injection when injected intrathecally in rabbits. Read before the Research Council of the Long Beach Memorial Hospital Medical Center, Long Beach, Calif., June 1969.

Woessner J.F. Jr.: Enzymatic mechanisms for the degradation of connective tissue matrix, in Owen P., Godfellow J., Bullough P. (eds.): *Orthopaedics and Traumatology*. London, William Heinemann Med. Books, Ltd., 1980, pp. 391–400.
[*Proposes a theory for the biochemical basis of osteoarthritis.*]

Wolf S.: Effects of suggestion and conditioning on the action of chemical agents in human subjects: The pharmacology of placebos. *J. Clin. Invest.* 29:100, 1950.

Wolf S., Pinsky R.H.: Effects of placebo administration and occurrence of toxic reactions. *JAMA* 155:339, 1954.

Wollin D.G., Lamon G.B., Cawley A.J., et al.: Neurotoxic effect of water soluble contrast media in spinal canal with emphasis on appropriate management. *J. Can. Assoc. Radiol.* 18:296, 1967.

Woodhall B.: The study of ground substance in intervertebral disc degeneration, abstracted. *J. Bone Joint Surg.* 36-A:1112, 1954.

World Medical Association: Declaration of Helsinki: Recommendations guiding doctors in clinical research. *JAMA* 197:31, 1966.

Young H.H.: Non-neurological lesions simulating protruded intervertebral disk. *JAMA* 148:1101, 1952.

Zaleske D.J., Ehrlich M.G., Huddleston J.I. Jr.: Combined biochemical and clinical investigation of chemonucleolysis failures. *Clin. Orthop.* 126:121, 1977.

Zwieman B., Hildreth E.: An approach to the performance of contrast studies in contrast material: Reactive persons. *Ann. Intern. Med.* 83:159, 1975.

COLOR PLATES

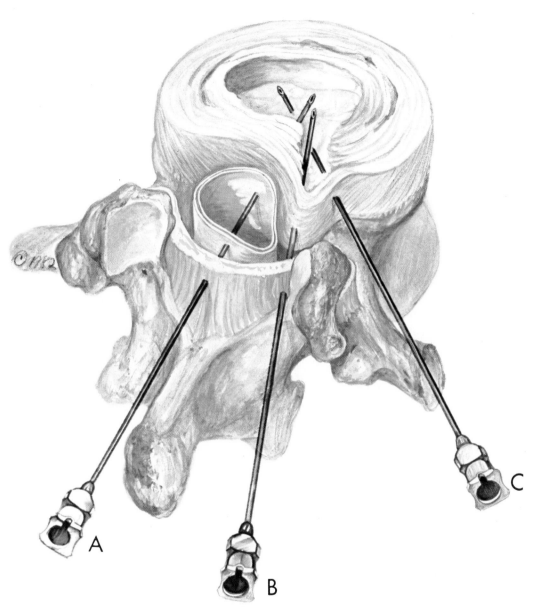

Plate 1.—Approaches to intradiscal injection. *A,* transdural (Lindblom). *B,* poster-olateral (Erlacher).[20] *C,* lateral (Edholm).[23]

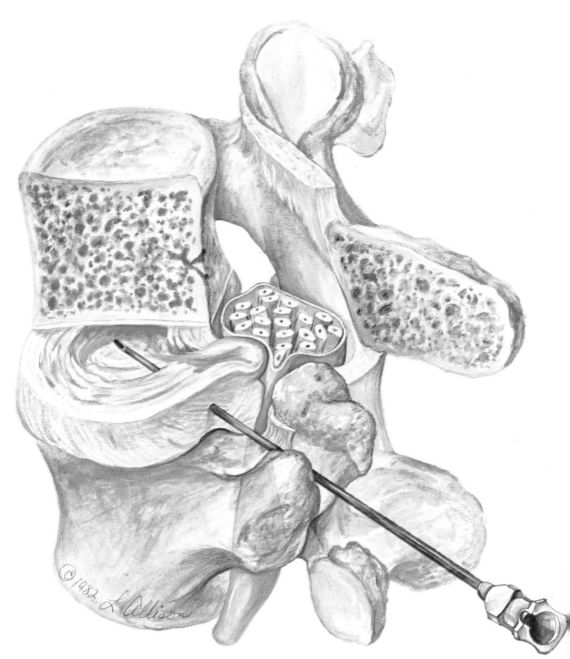

Plate 2.—Needle is inserted on the side of the disc herniation and leg pain.

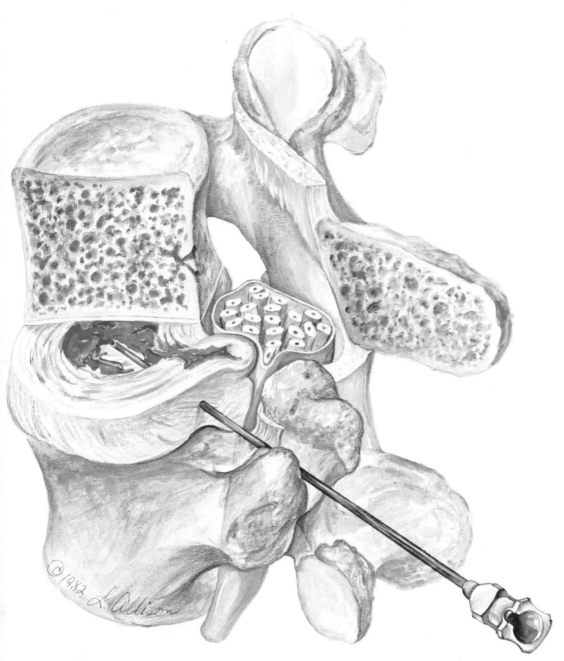

Plate 3.—After injecting contrast dye or enzyme, the area of extradural defect noted on the myelogram should fill up. Note the flow pattern of dye into herniated nucleus pulposus.

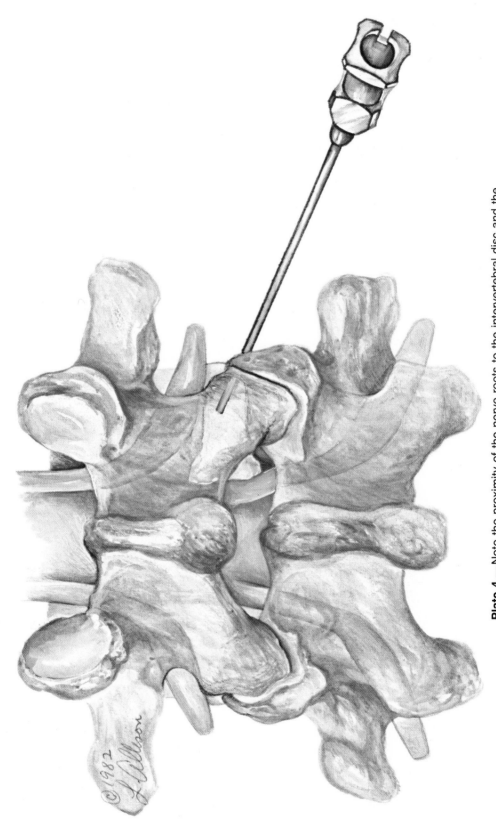

Plate 4.—Note the proximity of the nerve roots to the intervertebral disc and the point of insertion of the needle into the posterior lateral corner of the disc, as seen from a posterior view.

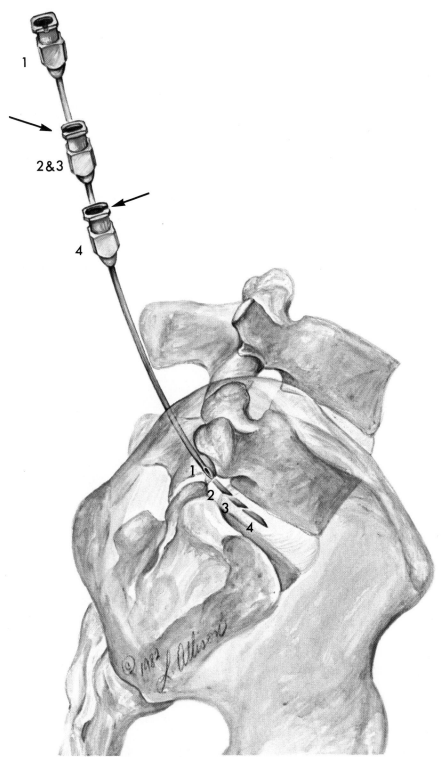

Plate 5.—Notch on the needle hub faces laterally, with the opening of the needle (lateral position 1) at the pars interarticularis. At positions 2 and 3, the bevel of the needle faces inferiorly, and the needle is directed around the corner toward the center of the disc space. At position 4 (the final point of insertion into the center of the disc), the bevel is turned superiorly. Note the notch on the hub *(arrow),* position 4.

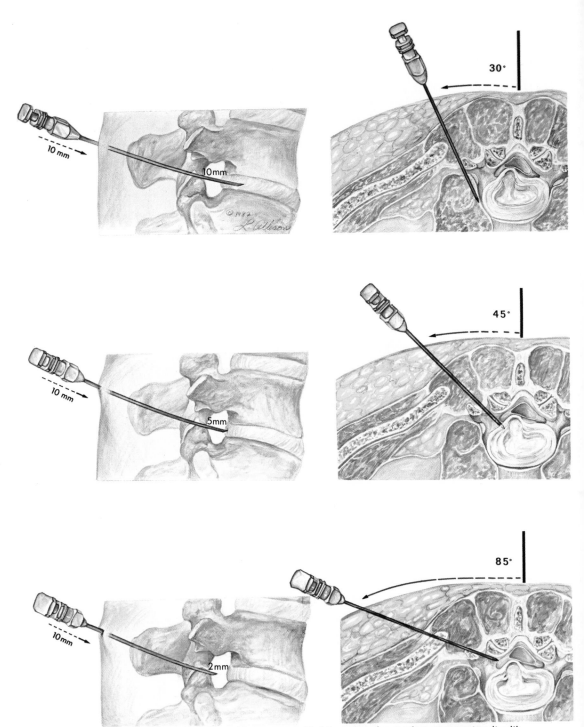

Plate 6.—Lateral *(left)* and transverse *(right)* views of a motion segment unit with needle insertion. *Top,* angle of needle insertion is too small with respect to the sagittal plane. On reaching the facet joint and pars interarticularis in the lateral fluoroscopic view, 10 mm of insertion of the needle into the skin will appear as 10 mm on the fluoroscopy screen. *Middle,* when the angle is correct, 10 mm of insertion will equal 5 mm on the screen. *Bottom,* when the angle with the sagittal plane is too large, insertion of the needle 1 cm into the skin will show very little further advancement of the needle on the lateral fluoroscopic view.

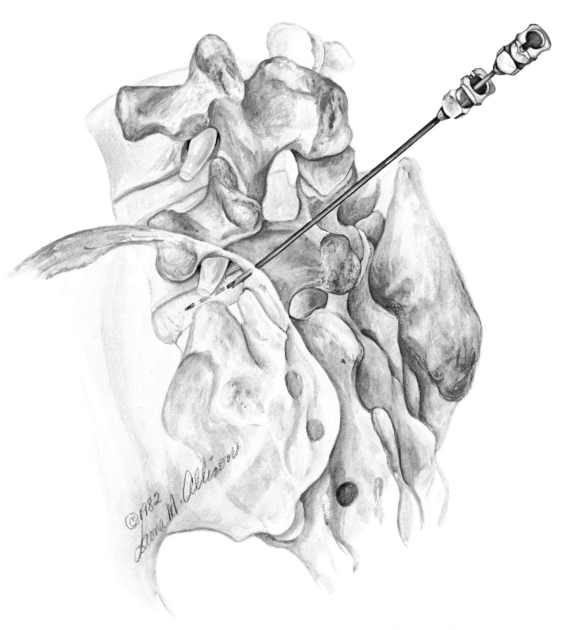

Plate 7.—The double-needle technique with an 18-gauge needle inserted into the posterior lateral corner of the lumbosacral disc and a 22-gauge needle inserted into the disc with the bevel faced laterally.

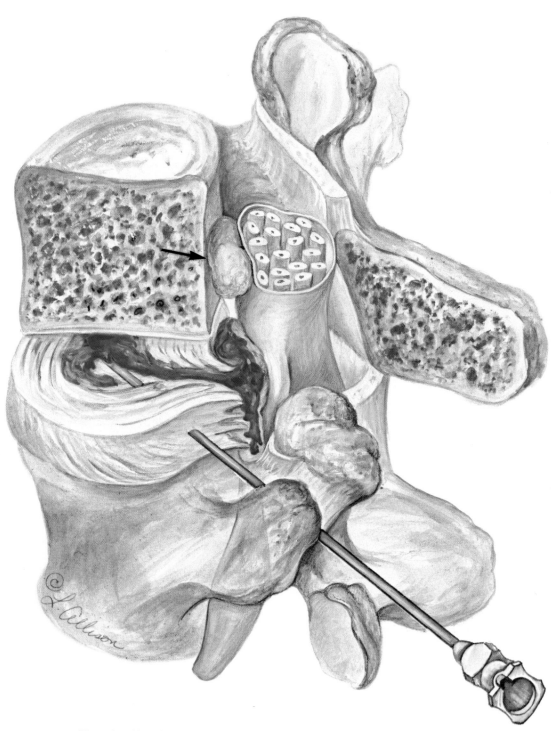

Plate 8.—Note how the intradiscally injected enzyme *(dark area)* flows into the extruded disc fragment but is not imbibed by the sequestrated fragment posterior to the sagittally sectioned vertebral body.

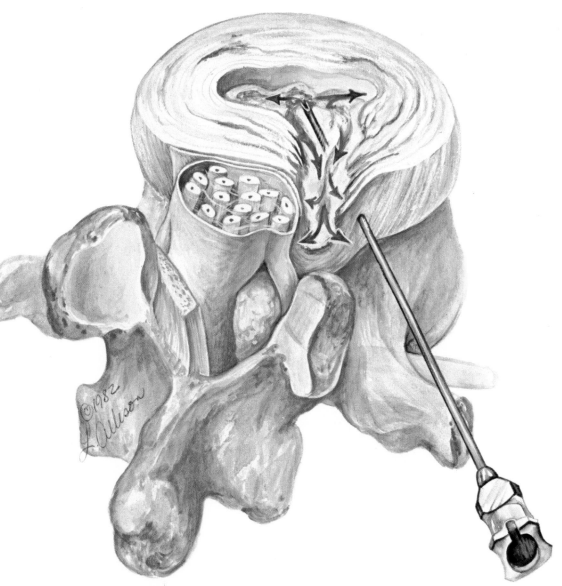

Plate 9.—The enzyme was effective in dissolving the central nucleus pulposus and leaked into the epidural space *(arrows),* but at surgery a large sequestrated fragment of disc was found in axilla of a nerve root.

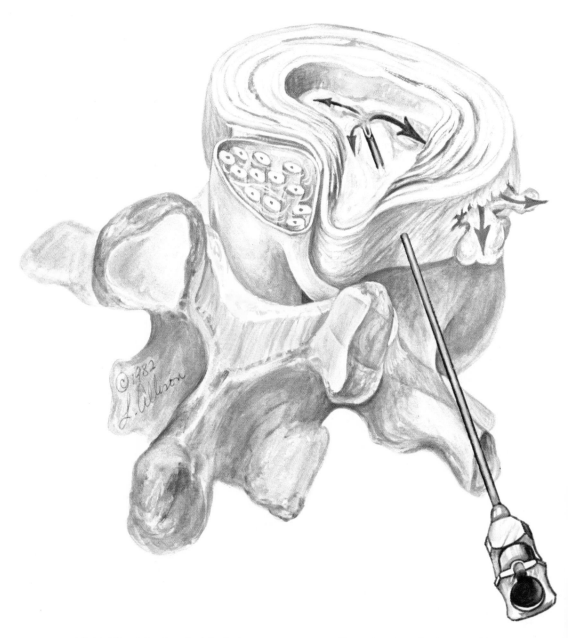

Plate 10.—Intradiscally injected enzyme escapes through a tear in the annulus away from the clinically significant posterolateral disc protrusion *(arrows).* This is an example of the enzyme taking the path of least resistance and may explain some failures of the technique.

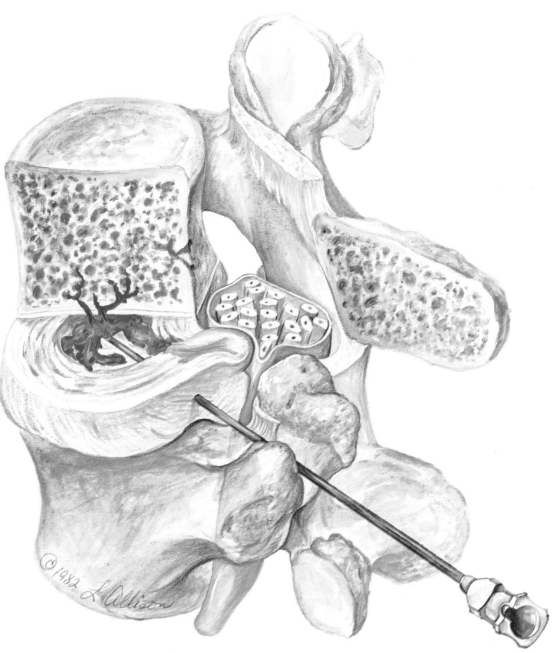

Plate 11.—Intradiscally injected enzyme *(dark area at tip of needle)* takes a path of least resistance through a crack in the bony end plate into the subchondral vascular channels. The clinically significant disc protrusion does not imbibe the enzyme.

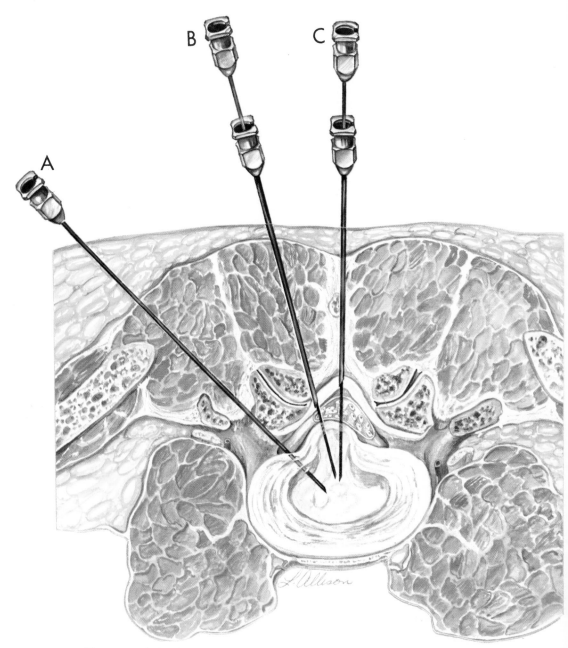

Plate 12.—Cross-section of the lumbosacral disc with the two-needle technique for injection by the lateral approach *(A)*, the posterolateral approach *(B)*, and the midline approach *(C)*. The lateral approach *(A)* is the only permissible route for intradiscal injection.